Closing Evidence Gaps in Clinical Prevention

Alexis Wojtowicz, Kathleen Stratton, and Tracy A. Lieu, *Editors*

Committee on Addressing Evidence Gaps in
Clinical Prevention Recommendations

Board on Population Health and Public Health Practice

Health and Medicine Division

A Consensus Study Report of

The National Academies of
SCIENCES · ENGINEERING · MEDICINE

THE NATIONAL ACADEMIES PRESS
Washington, DC
www.nap.edu

THE NATIONAL ACADEMIES PRESS 500 Fifth Street, NW Washington, DC 20001

This activity was supported with federal funds from the Agency for Healthcare Research and Quality and the National Institutes of Health, U.S. Department of Health and Human Services, Contract/Task Order No. HHSN263201800029I/75N98020F00005. Any opinions, findings, conclusions, or recommendations expressed in this publication do not necessarily reflect the views of any organization or agency that provided support for the project.

International Standard Book Number-13: 978-0-309-26957-5
International Standard Book Number-10: 0-309-26957-1
Digital Object Identifier: https://doi.org/10.17226/26351
Library of Congress Catalog Number: 2021951344

Additional copies of this publication are available from the National Academies Press, 500 Fifth Street, NW, Keck 360, Washington, DC 20001; (800) 624-6242 or (202) 334-3313; http://www.nap.edu.

Printed in the United States of America

Suggested citation: National Academies of Sciences, Engineering, and Medicine. 2022. *Closing evidence gaps in clinical prevention*. Washington, DC: The National Academies Press. https://doi.org/10.17226/26351.

The National Academies of

SCIENCES • ENGINEERING • MEDICINE

The **National Academy of Sciences** was established in 1863 by an Act of Congress, signed by President Lincoln, as a private, nongovernmental institution to advise the nation on issues related to science and technology. Members are elected by their peers for outstanding contributions to research. Dr. Marcia McNutt is president.

The **National Academy of Engineering** was established in 1964 under the charter of the National Academy of Sciences to bring the practices of engineering to advising the nation. Members are elected by their peers for extraordinary contributions to engineering. Dr. John L. Anderson is president.

The **National Academy of Medicine** (formerly the Institute of Medicine) was established in 1970 under the charter of the National Academy of Sciences to advise the nation on medical and health issues. Members are elected by their peers for distinguished contributions to medicine and health. Dr. Victor J. Dzau is president.

The three Academies work together as the **National Academies of Sciences, Engineering, and Medicine** to provide independent, objective analysis and advice to the nation and conduct other activities to solve complex problems and inform public policy decisions. The National Academies also encourage education and research, recognize outstanding contributions to knowledge, and increase public understanding in matters of science, engineering, and medicine.

Learn more about the National Academies of Sciences, Engineering, and Medicine at **www.nationalacademies.org**.

COMMITTEE ON ADDRESSING EVIDENCE GAPS IN CLINICAL PREVENTION RECOMMENDATIONS

TRACY A. LIEU (*Chair*), Director of the Division of Research, Kaiser Permanente Northern California
CATHY J. BRADLEY, Professor and Associate Dean for Research, Colorado School of Public Health; Deputy Director, University of Colorado Cancer Center
THEODORE G. GANIATS, Professor Emeritus, Department of Family Medicine and Public Health, University of California, San Diego, School of Medicine
KENG-YEN HUANG, Associate Professor, Departments of Population Health and Child & Adolescent Psychiatry, New York University Grossman School of Medicine
PREETI GOKAL KOCHAR, Technical Information Specialist, National Library of Medicine, National Institutes of Health
ANN E. KURTH, Dean and Linda Koch Lorimer Professor of Nursing, Yale School of Nursing; Professor of Epidemiology of Microbial Diseases, Yale School of Public Health
TIANJING LI, Associate Professor, Department of Ophthalmology, University of Colorado School of Medicine
K. M. VENKAT NARAYAN, Director, Emory Global Diabetes Research Center; Ruth and O.C. Hubert Chair of Global Health and Professor of Epidemiology, Rollins School of Public Health; Professor of Medicine, Emory University School of Medicine
WANDA K. NICHOLSON, Professor, Department of General Obstetrics & Gynecology and Director, Diabetes and Obesity Core Center for Women's Health Research, University of North Carolina School of Medicine
ELIZABETH O. OFILI, Professor of Medicine, Morehouse School of Medicine; Chief Medical Officer, Morehouse Choice Accountable Care Organization
NICOLAAS P. PRONK, President and Chief Science Officer, HealthPartners Institute
ROBERT B. WALLACE, Irene Ensminger Stecher Professor Emeritus of Epidemiology and Internal Medicine, University of Iowa College of Public Health

Study Staff

KATHLEEN R. STRATTON, Study Director
ALEXIS WOJTOWICZ, Associate Program Officer
AYSHIA COLETRANE, Senior Program Assistant
REBECCA MORGAN, Senior Librarian
MISRAK DABI, Finance Business Partner
ROSE MARIE MARTINEZ, Senior Board Director

Science Writer

ROBERT POOL

Reviewers

This Consensus Study Report was reviewed in draft form by individuals chosen for their diverse perspectives and technical expertise. The purpose of this independent review is to provide candid and critical comments that will assist the National Academies of Sciences, Engineering, and Medicine in making each published report as sound as possible and to ensure that it meets the institutional standards for quality, objectivity, evidence, and responsiveness to the study charge. The review comments and draft manuscript remain confidential to protect the integrity of the deliberative process.

We thank the following individuals for their review of this report:

SARABETH BRODER-FINGERT, University of Massachusetts
ROGER CHOU, Oregon Health & Science University
LAWRENCE S. B. GOLDSTEIN, University of California, San Diego
DAVID GROSSMAN, Kaiser Permanente
RICHARD M. HOFFMAN, University of Iowa
RANDY A. JONES, University of Virginia
ALEX KRIST, Virginia Commonwealth University
DONALD R. MATTISON, University of South Carolina
MARIA MORA PINZON, Wisconsin Alzheimer's Institute
HEIDI D. NELSON, Oregon Health & Science University
JOHN E. NIEDERHUBER, Johns Hopkins University

DOUG K. OWENS, Stanford University
JOE SELBY, Patient-Centered Outcomes Research Institute (retired)
STEPHANIE ZAZA, Centers for Disease Control and Prevention (retired)

Although the reviewers listed above provided many constructive comments and suggestions, they were not asked to endorse the content of the report nor did they see the final draft before its release. The review of this report was overseen by **BOBBIE BERKOWITZ,** Columbia University, and **JACK EBELER,** Health Policy Alternatives, Inc. They were responsible for making certain that an independent examination of this report was carried out in accordance with standards of the National Academies and that all review comments were carefully considered. Responsibility for the final content rests entirely with the authoring committee and the National Academies.

Preface

Preventing suffering and loss of life through early identification and treatment of individuals at risk is a central purpose of clinical care. For decades, primary care clinicians and others have relied on recommendations of the U.S. Preventive Services Task Force (USPSTF) in these efforts. The USPSTF's careful reliance on evidence from rigorous studies to inform its statements has often highlighted topics and questions for which the evidence is insufficient to make a definitive recommendation. In an ideal world, when an insufficient evidence statement is rendered, research sponsors and researchers should quickly initiate high-quality studies needed to fill the most important evidence gaps. However, in some cases the lack of a widely agreed-on framework for describing and categorizing such evidence gaps has hampered efficient communication and progress.

The present study focused on developing a taxonomy to characterize evidence gaps in clinical prevention, and identifying research strategies and funding approaches to enable sponsors and researchers to more effectively fill these gaps. This work was sponsored by leaders in the National Institutes of Health (NIH) and the Agency for Healthcare Research and Quality (AHRQ), which supports the USPSTF. We are grateful to David Murray and Carrie Klabunde of the Office of Disease Prevention, NIH, and to Arlene Bierman and Amanda Borsky of the Center for Evidence and Practice Improvement, AHRQ, for their guidance and support. We also wish to acknowledge the important contributions of Susan Curry, who was instrumental in launching this effort.

Our study committee approached this task with a sense of significance and optimism, and demonstrated intellectual generosity and graciousness throughout this multidisciplinary process. The committee and the Health and Medicine Division's (HMD's) staff of the National Academies developed this report and the taxonomy in an iterative manner, based on reviews of existing USPSTF recommendation statements and public meetings with experts from NIH, AHRQ, and other key organizations that sponsor research or support guideline committees, USPSTF members, and the research community. During this process we were particularly attuned to the fact that both the USPSTF and research sponsors must balance competing priorities among the many evidence gaps that could be addressed. As a former member of the USPSTF, the past chair of an NIH grant review committee, and a leader of a research department in a health care delivery system, I greatly appreciated the ability of our committee members and expert key informants to think pragmatically about how to facilitate communication and collaboration by the multiple stakeholders needed to successfully address evidence gaps.

We appreciate the education offered us by the speakers at our public meetings, including the following:

- **David Atkins, M.D., M.P.H.,** *Director,* Health Services Research & Development, U.S. Department of Veterans Affairs
- **Arlene Bierman, M.D., M.S.,** *Director,* Center for Evidence and Practice Improvement, AHRQ
- **Amanda Borsky, Dr.P.H., M.P.P.,** *Program Manager,* USPSTF, AHRQ
- **Sarabeth Broder-Fingert, M.D., M.P.H.,** *Associate Professor of Pediatrics,* Boston University School of Medicine; *Co-Director,* Innovation in Autism Disparities, Inclusion, Outreach, and Transition Services Lab, Boston University
- **Ned Calonge, M.D., M.P.H.,** *President and Chief Executive Officer,* Colorado Trust; *Associate Professor of Family Medicine,* Colorado School of Medicine, and *Associate Professor of Epidemiology,* Colorado School of Public Health, University of Colorado Denver
- **Doug Corley, M.D., Ph.D.,** *Lead Investigator,* National Cancer Institute (NCI) Population-based Research to Optimize the Screening Process Consortium; *Research Scientist,* Kaiser Permanente Northern California Division of Research
- **Susan Curry, Ph.D.,** *Senior Advisor for Preventive Services,* NIH; *Dean Emerita and Distinguished Professor of Health Management and Policy,* University of Iowa

- **Paul Doria-Rose, Ph.D., D.V.M.,** *Chief,* Healthcare Assessment Research Branch, Health Delivery Research Program, Division of Cancer Control & Population Sciences, NCI
- **Chyke Doubeni, M.D., M.P.H.,** *Member,* USPSTF; *Director,* Mayo Clinic Center for Health Equity and Community Engagement Research
- **Carrie Klabunde, Ph.D.,** *Senior Advisor for Disease Prevention,* Office of Disease Prevention, NIH
- **Alex Krist, M.D., M.P.H.,** *Immediate Past Chair,* USPSTF; *Professor of Family Medicine and Population Health,* Virginia Commonwealth University
- **Amy Lansky, Ph.D., M.P.H.,** *Director,* Centers for Disease Control and Prevention Community Guide
- **Michael Lauer, M.D.,** *Deputy Director,* Extramural Research, NIH
- **Alan Leshner, Ph.D.,** *Chief Executive Officer Emeritus,* American Association for the Advancement of Science; *Executive Publisher, Science; Former Director,* National Institute on Drug Abuse, NIH; *Former Deputy Director and Acting Director,* National Institute of Mental Health (NIMH), NIH
- **Carol Mangione, M.D., M.S.P.H., FACP,** *Vice-Chair,* USPSTF; *Chief,* Division of General Medicine & Health Services Research, University of California, Los Angeles (UCLA); *Barbara A. Levey & Gerald S. Levey Professor of Medicine and Public Health,* UCLA
- **David Murray, Ph.D.,** *Associate Director for Prevention* and *Director,* Office of Disease Prevention, NIH
- **Karen Robinson, Ph.D., M.Sc.,** *Director,* Evidence-based Practice Center, Johns Hopkins University
- **Michael Silverstein, M.D., M.P.H.,** *Member,* USPSTF; *Professor of Pediatrics, Director,* Division of General Academic Pediatrics, and *Vice Chair,* Research for the Department of Pediatrics, Boston University School of Medicine
- **Harold (Hal) Sox, M.D.,** *Director,* Peer Review, Patient-Centered Outcomes Research Institute
- **Ann Wagner, Ph.D.,** *National Autism Coordinator,* Office of NIMH Director, NIMH, NIH

We are also grateful to Caitlin Phelps (American College of Obstetricians and Gynecologists), Joe Selby, Steve Teutsch, and Gregory Traversy (Public Health Agency of Canada) for their helpful observations and suggestions.

The committee's work would not have been possible without the insightful leadership of our study director Kathleen Stratton and the thoughtful and analytic contributions of Associate Program Officer Alexis

Wojtowicz. We benefited from the excellent organizational skills of Ayshia Coletrane and the lucid writing assistance of Robert Pool as we crafted this report. We extend thanks to Rose Marie Martinez for her farsighted guidance and to the National Academies' Research Center staff and many other staff members within HMD and the National Academies for their support.

The committee hopes this study will facilitate a common understanding of the key concepts related to evidence gaps in clinical prevention, support thoughtful discussion of priorities among multiple stakeholders, and lead to research that enhances clinical prevention in the years ahead.

Tracy A. Lieu, *Chair*
Committee on Addressing Evidence Gaps
in Clinical Prevention Recommendations

Contents

Boxes, Figures, and Tables

BOXES

FIGURES

TABLES

Acronyms and Abbreviations

AAA	abdominal aortic aneurysm
ACA	Patient Protection and Affordable Care Act
ACE	angiotensin-converting enzyme
AHCPR	Agency for Healthcare Policy and Research
AHRQ	Agency for Healthcare Research and Quality
ASD	autism spectrum disorder
CDC	Centers for Disease Control and Prevention
CDMRP	Congressionally Directed Medical Research Program
CISNET	Cancer Intervention and Surveillance Modeling Network
CPG	clinical practice guideline
CPSTF	Community Preventive Services Task Force
CT	computed tomography
CTFPHE	Canadian Task Force on the Public Health Examination
CTSA	Clinical and Translational Science Awards
D&I	dissemination and implementation
DOD	U.S. Department of Defense
ECG	electrocardiography
EPC	Evidence-based Practice Center

FIT	fecal immunochemical testing
FOA	funding opportunity announcement
FY	fiscal year
HHS	U.S. Department of Health and Human Services
HMD	Health and Medicine Division
HRSA	Health Resources and Services Administration
IC	institutes and centers
MCI	mild cognitive impairment
NCI	National Cancer Institute
NHLBI	National Heart, Lung, and Blood Institute
NIH	National Institutes of Health
NIMH	National Institute of Mental Health
NOSI	notice of special interest
ODP	Office of Disease Prevention
PA	program announcement
PCORI	Patient-Centered Outcomes Research Institute
PICO	population, intervention, comparison, outcomes
PICOTS	population, intervention, comparison, outcome, timing, setting
PRC	Prevention Research Center
PrEP	preexposure prophylaxis
PROSPR	Population-based Research to Optimize the Screening Process
RCT	randomized controlled trial
RFA	request for application
RFP	request for proposal
SBIR	Small Business Innovation Research
SBTT	Small Business Technology Transfer
SPRINT	Systolic Blood Pressure Intervention Trial
SVS	Society for Vascular Surgery
UCLA	University of California, Los Angeles
USPSTF	U.S. Preventive Services Task Force
VA	U.S. Department of Veterans Affairs

Summary

In 1984, the U.S. Department of Health and Human Services (HHS) assistant secretary Edward N. Brandt commissioned the U.S. Preventive Services Task Force (USPSTF) to "improve the health of people nationwide by making evidence-based recommendations about clinical preventive services" (USPSTF, n.d.). The USPSTF was assembled as an effort to continue and expand the innovative work of the Canadian Task Force on the Periodic Health Examination (CTFPHE) within the United States (CTFPHE, 1979; McGinnis and Woolf, 1990). The CTFPHE laid out the basic elements of clinical preventive evidence assessment as they inform clinical practice guidelines (CPGs). These included comprehensively reviewing the literature; using prioritization methods for assessing individual interventions, including determining the burden of suffering and ability to measure outcomes; understanding the risks and benefits of an intervention; rating the effectiveness of interventions; grading the level of evidence for a recommendation; and defining a research agenda to address unanswered questions (CTFPHE, 1979). The USPSTF is codified in the Healthcare Research and Quality Act, which states that the USPSTF

> shall review the scientific evidence related to the effectiveness, appropriateness, and cost-effectiveness of clinical preventive services for the

purpose of developing recommendations for the health care community, and updating previous clinical preventive recommendations.[1]

However, despite having the authority to do so, the USPSTF does not evaluate evidence related to cost-effectiveness when issuing a grade for a topic:

> [USPSTF] excludes costs from its determination of the benefits and harms of a clinical preventive service. This deliberate decision was made to maintain a clear focus on the science of clinical effectiveness (i.e., "what works"), and not consider cost, in part to avoid any misperception that the Task Force's purpose is to limit health care based on cost.... The Task Force recognizes that cost is a consideration for insurers, health systems, purchasers, and consumers. The USPSTF maintains that regardless of how health care is financed, it is essential to understand what the science says about which preventive services work. (USPSTF, 2021c)

The USPSTF recommendations guide clinical practice and garner broad attention, as evidenced by the coverage in the lay and medical literature of the recent change in guidance regarding aspirin use to prevent cardiovascular disease (Mahase, 2021; Rabin, 2021; USPSTF, 2021a).

The USPSTF's process of selecting a topic for review through publishing the final recommendation statement takes 3 years on average (Borsky, 2021). The USPSTF works with one of the Evidence-based Practice Centers (EPCs) supported by the Agency for Healthcare Research and Quality (AHRQ) to develop a draft research plan, which is posted for public comment. After the USPSTF and the EPC review and revise as needed, the final plan is posted online. The EPC conducts the evidence review according to the research plan, and the USPSTF begins assessing the EPC's draft review. The USPSTF then drafts a recommendation statement, posts it online for, and reviews any public comments, and the EPC finalizes its evidence review. The USPSTF then finalizes its recommendation statement, and both are posted online and, as of 2016, published in a journal of the JAMA Network (Bauchner et al., 2016). The USPSTF also considers previously graded topics for updates starting 2–3 years after they are first published, soliciting stakeholder input and examining the likelihood that enough new evidence has been developed that the recommendation for practice may be updated.

The USPSTF assessment of the overall evidence for a clinical preventive service requires two key determinations: assessment of the degree

[1] 106th U.S. Congress, First Session. Public Law 106-129, Section 915. Healthcare Research and Quality Act of 1999. https://www.ahrq.gov/sites/default/files/wysiwyg/policymakers/hrqa99.pdf (accessed July 20, 2021).

of certainty about the net benefit (benefits minus harms) and assessment of the magnitude of net benefit for the population for whom the service is intended. Currently, the USPSTF recommends offering or providing preventive services with grades A or B; selectively offering or providing a preventive service with a grade C; and *not* offering or providing a preventive service with a grade D. While the recommendations for or against a clinical service receive a grade, some topics are given I statements, indicating that the USPSTF has not found sufficient evidence to make a recommendation at all. In 2009, the USPSTF announced that it would use the term "I statement" instead of "I recommendation" to reduce confusion among clinicians about the fact that an I statement was not a recommendation (USPSTF, 2017). Topics can receive an I statement instead of a graded recommendation due to lack of evidence, a lack of good-quality evidence, or an abundance of conflicting evidence. As of publication of this report, 53 of 86 published topics have I statements either for a specific subpopulation or for recommending for or against the service at all. The USPSTF has suggested evidence gaps or research needs related to the statement topic since its first report, though a 2019 methods update formalized a Research Needs and Gaps section for each statement. Both I statements and letter grade recommendations include research needs; the details of those sections vary widely in their specificity and scope. Addressing evidence gaps is important for changing an I statement to a letter grade recommendation or, as in the case of the recent change in the draft recommendation regarding aspirin use to prevent cardiovascular disease, changing a letter grade recommendation, in this example from a C recommendation to a D for some populations (USPSTF, 2021a).

STATEMENT OF TASK

An ad hoc committee of the National Academies of Sciences, Engineering, and Medicine (the National Academies) was convened to examine current issues in identifying and filling evidence gaps in the USPSTF clinical prevention recommendations. The committee was specifically tasked with developing a taxonomy of evidence gaps. The complete Statement of Task can be found in Chapter 1. At the first meeting of the committee, David Murray, the director of the Office of Disease Prevention (ODP) at the National Institutes of Health (NIH), characterized the challenges in addressing evidence gaps in two ways: nonspecific descriptions (e.g., "high-quality studies on the potential harms of screening and treatment are needed") and discussion of evidence gaps in various places. Expressly stated was the hope to link evidence gaps with USPSTF criteria for study inclusion and coordinated effort to describe and communicate evidence gaps so that they are easier to identify and address (Murray,

2020). Thus, AHRQ and ODP expressed a desire for a more systematic way for the USPSTF and NIH to work together to describe research needs and make them more actionable. Both AHRQ and ODP representatives stressed that the audience for the report is not limited to the USPSTF, AHRQ, or NIH—rather, it is hoped that the report would be helpful to CPG developers, research funders, and researchers.

Committee Process

The committee held four open sessions to solicit input on the Statement of Task, experiences of others in developing taxonomies, and challenges for NIH and researchers to address I statements. The committee reviewed literature on taxonomies and developed a taxonomy using current I statements as test candidates for the taxonomy. As part of its work, the committee developed a workflow to show how to use the taxonomy to develop a research agenda.

TAXONOMY

Taxonomies come in various forms, but they all share certain characteristics. The general purpose of any taxonomy is to bring order to a collection of information by organizing and systematizing it, often with a fixed vocabulary and clearly defined structure. A well-designed taxonomy makes it easier to see the big picture and to think about and work with the mass of information that it has imposed order on. The taxonomy adopted by the committee provides a systematic way of describing evidence gaps with a clear list of categories and a controlled vocabulary for consistency across evidence reviews. Furthermore, by offering a list of the different classes of evidence gaps that may play a role in analyzing a preventive service, the taxonomy and an accompanying workflow offer a road map for researchers and funders.

The USPSTF analytic framework begins with the specification of a population of interest and then examines the evidence for connections between actions (screening, preventive medications, or behavioral interventions) and outcomes (early detection, decreased morbidity or mortality, adverse effects) (see Figure S-1). Each line in the figure between an action and an outcome is associated with a question of interest: Does screening lead to an early detection of the target condition? Does screening lead to adverse effects? Do early detection and treatment lead to reduced morbidity or mortality? Do early detection and treatment lead to an intermediate outcome that may in turn be related to a decrease in morbidity or mortality? Do early detection and treatment lead to adverse effects? When the USPSTF examines the evidence concerning the effectiveness of

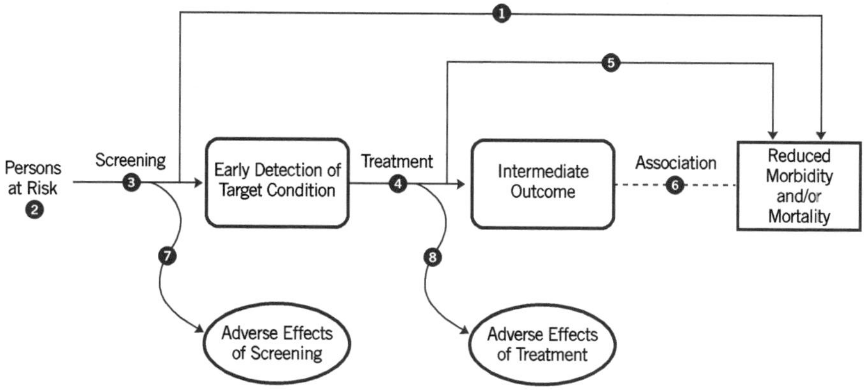

FIGURE S-1 A generic version of the analytic framework used by the U.S. Preventive Services Task Force.
SOURCE: USPSTF, 2021b.

a particular preventive service, it uses these particular questions to guide its analysis and to frame the reporting of its results. It should also be noted that while this generic framework focuses specifically on screenings, the USPSTF uses this approach to guide its recommendations for preventive medications and behavioral counseling as well (see Chapter 4 for more varied and complex examples of the USPSTF analytic frameworks).

The committee realized that these various pieces of the analytic framework—such as the population under consideration, early detection, intermediate outcomes, effectiveness, harms—could serve as a good starting point for a taxonomy for characterizing the various research needs and other issues associated with a given preventive service. However, they determined that a taxonomy consisting only of elements from the analytic framework would be incomplete, and thus they added other components.

One set of missing elements could be classified as foundational issues, such as a lack of clarity on nomenclature or on the specificity of a screening tool. Another set of issues not touched upon in the USPSTF analytic framework involves the dissemination and implementation (D&I) of a recommended preventive service. Traditionally this has not been something that the USPSTF has concerned itself with, but the committee's discussions led it to conclude that it was crucial to include evidence gaps related to D&I in the taxonomy.

Thus, the committee developed a taxonomy that covers three different facets of prevention-related evidence gaps: foundational issues, clinical and epidemiologic evidence as outlined in the USPSTF's analytic framework, and D&I. The committee also wanted the taxonomy to be useful for outlining a prioritized research agenda. Thus, the committee offers a taxonomy for use in prioritizing research gaps as well as a way to specify the types of studies needed to fill those gaps. All terms are expanded and defined in Chapter 4, which also includes two examples of applying the evidence gap taxonomy to two recent I statements issued by the USPSTF. See Figure S-2 for the basic workflow to use with the taxonomy terms; the complete workflow can be found in Chapter 4. In addition to the taxonomy itself, a workflow guiding users through using each facet of the taxonomy can be found in Chapter 4.

Per the workflow, the first step is to review the evidence concerning a particular preventive service in order to develop a recommendation statement. As described in the recommendations, the evidence base may be insufficient to answer certain questions, and in those cases, it will be necessary to gather additional information from stakeholders.

Once the review of evidence has been completed, the next step is to use the taxonomy to identify the gaps that exist in the evidence. These gaps will be placed in one of three facets: foundational issues, analytic framework evidence gaps, and D&I evidence gaps. Generally speaking, any gaps that would leave a topic with an I statement would be put into one of the first two facets; that is, those two facets cover the evidence gaps that have traditionally been considered by the USPSTF.

After identifying and characterizing any evidence gaps using the first three facets of the taxonomy, users will develop a research agenda using two additional facets. Users will prioritize evidence gaps within the topic being reviewed using criteria from the prioritization facet, clarifying which evidence gaps are most important to address, so limited research funding can be put to optimal use. Users will then use the study specification facet to outline the important aspects of the key research studies needed to address the high-priority evidence gaps. The study specification facet is an expansion of the PICOTS (population, intervention, comparison, outcome, timing, setting) framework.

Not every interested party will necessarily carry out every step in the framework. Some might, for example, choose to focus on the traditional USPSTF concerns and apply only the first two parts of the taxonomy—covering foundational issues and analytic framework issues—and not address D&I. Others, such as funders, might work with a collection of evidence gaps generated by someone else and apply their own prioritization criteria to develop a research agenda that reflects their own interests.

RECOMMENDATIONS

The committee makes eight recommendations in three categories: using the taxonomy, fostering clinical prevention research, and advancing the work of the USPSTF. The committee's rationale follows each recommendation.

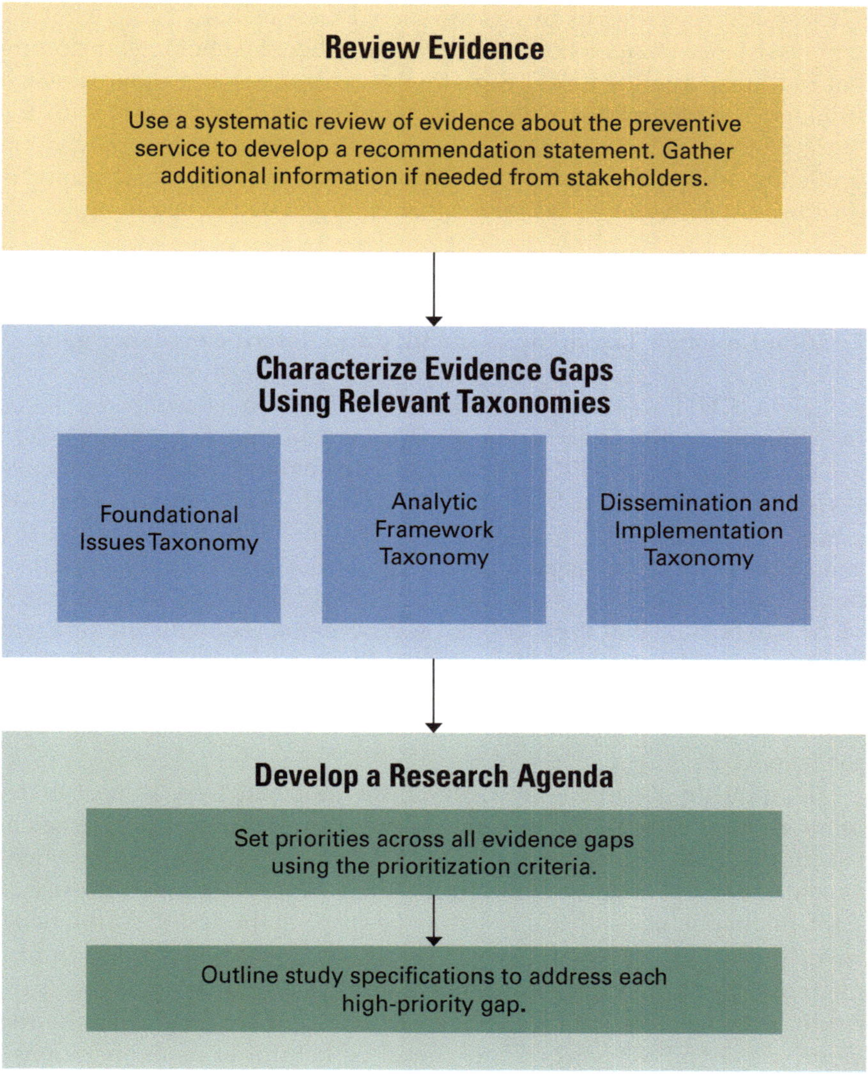

FIGURE S-2 Workflow for using the evidence gaps taxonomy.

Using the Taxonomy

The committee has provided a taxonomy for use in systematically describing evidence gaps in three facets: foundational research, the analytic framework used by the USPSTF, and D&I. The committee also outlines two additional facets to guide the process for developing a research agenda: prioritizing evidence gaps and outlining key research studies.

The committee envisions this as the shared responsibility of the USPSTF with assistance from AHRQ and ODP and other stakeholders, including but not limited to the USPSTF partner organizations and other research funders. The committee developed Recommendations 1 and 2 with the work of the USPSTF in mind but hopes that other clinical prevention guideline developers find this useful and adopt it. Recommendation 3 is directed at AHRQ and NIH to maintain and update the taxonomy.

Recommendation 1: For each of its recommendation statements, the U.S. Preventive Services Task Force should use the Clinical Prevention Research Taxonomy to identify and describe evidence gaps.

The USPSTF will likely and understandably be most inclined to focus their efforts on the analytic framework evidence gaps, as it is already a part of their process. These evidence gaps emerge from the evidence review provided by an EPC and the USPSTF deliberations about the grade recommendation (AHRQ, 2018). The USPSTF may also find the foundational evidence gaps facet useful, particularly because some recommendation and I statement Research Needs and Gaps sections name evidence gaps of that type, though not by name. Framing the research needs around the taxonomy terms will impart consistency in the USPSTF efforts to describe research needs. The committee envisions that AHRQ will direct EPCs to conduct reviews using terminology consistent with the taxonomy.

Despite the fact that the USPSTF has not had D&I as part of its remit, it recognizes the importance of D&I to clinical prevention research. Additionally, AHRQ has a robust portfolio on implementation research. Recently, USPSTF members and AHRQ staff wrote, "Although the use of implementation research is not within the scope of the USPSTF's deliberations, it notes that there are critical questions about how to best implement recommended clinical preventive services in primary care practices. Additional implementation and translational research will increase the value of the USPSTF's work and would be helpful in its deliberations" (Mabry-Hernandez et al., 2018, p. S98).

Because the committee was not tasked with recommending how the USPSTF determines its recommendations, it does not intend that D&I considerations would influence the letter grade recommendations issued by the USPSTF. However, it is clear from AHRQ's and ODP's request to the National Academies and the committee in open session that the committee was encouraged to address the clinical prevention community writ large and thus has proposed a D&I facet as part of the larger taxonomy of evidence gaps in clinical prevention (NASEM, 2020).

There are several ways the work related to D&I could be accomplished. The committee hopes that eventually the USPSTF will assume responsibility for D&I work; however, the committee understands that the USPSTF carries a large workload and that this requires time and resources to be fully implemented. In the short term, partner organizations and staff at AHRQ and NIH could provide pivotal support and input. D&I evidence gaps or questions might be similar for certain types of interventions. Attention to D&I might start with an effort to outline common themes or challenges to facilitate the work on specific I statements.

Recommendation 2: For each recommendation and I statement, the U.S. Preventive Services Task Force (USPSTF) should indicate high-priority evidence gaps. Staff from the Office of Disease Prevention (ODP) in the National Institutes of Health (NIH) and from the Agency for Healthcare Research and Quality (AHRQ) should broadly outline research that could address those priority gaps and be available to help funders, whether NIH or others, develop a research agenda to address them. The USPSTF and staff from ODP and AHRQ should consult partner organizations and stakeholders as needed.

The committee was urged to facilitate prioritizing the evidence gaps. In order to make those priorities evident and actionable by funders and researchers, the committee outlines two steps in the development of a research agenda: setting priorities across all evidence gaps and outlining key studies needed to address each high-priority evidence gap.

Given the demands on USPSTF members, the committee suggests that the development of a research agenda could be done by NIH and AHRQ staff in *consultation* with USPSTF members and stakeholders. If there are concerns about this process holding up issuance of a USPSTF recommendation statement, the research agenda could be published separately and subsequent to publication of the Recommendation statement itself. USPSTF members, however, are best suited to prioritize evidence gaps, especially regarding foundational research and analytic framework gaps. A structured approach to prioritization would be an important enhancement of the committee's work. Until that time, those prioritizing the evidence gaps can use the prioritization facet qualitatively or selectively. The USPSTF might initially focus on centrality or equity.

One of the frustrations identified by stakeholders is that the USPSTF research needs have not usually been specific enough with regard to some key elements of study design, such as whether a randomized controlled trial is required. As described in Chapter 4, the committee provides a taxonomy of study specifications based on an enhancement of the PICOTS framework for use by whomever completes the research agenda. The enhancements include aggregability, design considerations, and potential funders and funding mechanisms. The committee urges that the research agenda not be overly prescriptive, so as not to limit researcher creativity or funders' expectations of research proposals.

Recommendation 3: The National Institutes of Health and the Agency for Healthcare Research and Quality should make the taxonomy accessible on their websites and integrate the taxonomy terms and phrases in their relevant publications, including but not limited to U.S. Preventive Services Task Force recommendation statements, funding announcements, and grant and contract awards.

Consistent use of these metadata will provide a common language to stakeholders and encourage wider adoption of the taxonomy. Applying the taxonomy terms in publications linking USPSTF recommendations or I statements with funding opportunity announcements will be crucial for making evident the impact of the research agenda laid out by the USPSTF. In order to ensure relevance and usability, the taxonomy and workflow will need to be maintained, updated, and evaluated.

Fostering Clinical Prevention Research

The committee was asked to propose ways for prevention research funders and guideline developers to enhance their partnership to accelerate research to close important gaps in prevention. A robust and relevant clinical prevention research agenda requires funding, funding requests that are clear and clearly linked to USPSTF research needs, and appropriate mechanisms for and oversight of funded research. As such, the committee provides recommendations regarding the funding and commissioning of clinical prevention research.

Recommendation 4: Funders, in particular the National Institutes of Health and the Patient-Centered Outcomes Research Institute, should set aside funding to address high-priority evidence gaps identified by the U.S. Preventive Services Task Force.

In order to act in a timely manner on a research agenda for clinical prevention developed by the USPSTF, AHRQ staff and ODP and other NIH staff, EPCs, and other stakeholders, funding, especially dedicated funding, will be needed. NIH and stakeholders can work with Congress and HHS leadership to identify appropriate funding levels and secure sufficient funding for this area of need. Many research questions may require trans-institute collaboration, and these should be actively encouraged.

The committee acknowledges that calls for increased funding for prevention research have been made by others in the past and not always successfully. However, NIH's budget is approximately $41.7 billion, and in 2016 only 20 percent of that was, at best, spent on prevention research, broadly defined (Murray, 2017; NIH, 2020). The amount devoted to clinical prevention research of direct relevance to the USPSTF is undoubtedly much less.

Recommendation 5: The National Institutes of Health staff developing funding announcements for research related to high-priority evidence gaps should consult with the Office of Disease Prevention and the Agency for Healthcare Research and Quality to ensure appropriateness of support mechanisms and fidelity to the research specifications and should include a link to the research needs document on the U.S. Preventive Services Task Force website.

Program announcements, notices of special interest, requests for applications or proposals, and research opportunity announcements related to high-priority research needs of importance to the USPSTF should be as explicit as possible to ensure usefulness to the USPSTF and other guideline bodies. AHRQ and ODP staff could serve as an important resource in the crafting of the requests and notices. Reviewers of applications and proposals could be encouraged to study the research needs specification from the USPSTF. Study sections dedicated to these applications could ensure that study section members are oriented to the needs of the USPSTF.

Recommendation 6: The National Institutes of Health and other funders addressing high-priority clinical prevention evidence gaps identified by the U.S. Preventive Services Task Force should use funding mechanisms and processes that can assure that research is conducted expediently, efficiently, and with fidelity to the specified research needs, rather than waiting for such research needs to be addressed predominantly through investigator-initiated grant mechanisms.

A contract, or other directive funding mechanism increases the likelihood that studies are of sufficient design to allow for aggregating studies; to demonstrate an effect, if the intervention indeed is effective; and to meet the methodologic rigor for high-quality studies identified in USPSTF evidence syntheses. Consultation with the awardees regularly could ensure that the research is being conducted in a timely manner with fidelity to the research needs specification. Additionally, the committee encourages NIH and other funders to explore developing creative new programs that can be brought to bear on closing evidence gaps in clinical prevention. Expanding and establishing trans-NIH prevention interests into networks for clinical prevention research could also contribute to closing high-priority evidence gaps identified by the USPSTF by establishing an infrastructure to conduct prevention research. Such a network would complement the Centers for Disease Control and Prevention's Prevention Research Centers.

Advancing the Work of the USPSTF

The committee understands the immensity of the workload of the USPSTF, the rigor with which the members adhere to the advice of methodologists, and the importance of consistency of approach across time. The committee makes recommendations intended to enhance and advance the work of the USPSTF in order for them to provide as many definitive recommendations for practice as possible and to ensure that the recommendations lead to improved health of the target population.

Recommendation 7: The Agency for Healthcare Research and Quality should fund research in how guideline developers assess evidence and issue clinical practice guidelines, including how the decision of "insufficient evidence" is made and how a committee decides which research gaps are the key.

Most evidence-based CPGs include a statement of the level of the evidence and a separate statement on the strength of the recommendation. An evidence-based guideline may be explicit in terms of the methods for evaluating the level of evidence but not explicit in how the guideline committee uses many factors to determine not only the strength of the recommendation but the recommendation itself.

Different expert groups looking at the same topic can come up with different guideline statements. Sometimes this is because they look at different data (an accidentally incomplete literature review or a review that is purposefully limited by language, years of publication, study type). However, even if two guideline panels look at the same evidence there will often be differences in the guideline statements informed by differences in the *dynamics* of the guideline committee, different biases, and differences in the rules used for the guideline.

It is important to better understand the process of group decision making by a guideline panel. At times, how the committees works may be more important than the facts discussed. This means there are many questions on what determines which data the committee chooses to look at, how it evaluates the data, how it balances the different elements of the evidence, how the dynamics of the committee affect the final assessment/guideline statement, and so on. These questions, if addressed, can improve guideline fidelity and quality. Increasing the knowledge of the processes of group decision making may lead to methods for improving this task.

Recommendation 8: The Agency for Healthcare Research and Quality should work with relevant government agencies and key stakeholders to evaluate how effectively U.S. Preventive Services Task Force recommendations are implemented in real-world settings to identify and address gaps in achieving the intended benefits.

Simply making a recommendation may not have the intended impact on clinical care and population health. Evaluation of programs suggested by a recommendation can occur for both process and health outcomes. These evaluations ask if outcomes improve after the guideline is disseminated or implemented. For example, do colorectal cancer screenings increase after the guideline is published (process outcome); does colorectal cancer death decrease after the guideline is published (clinical outcome); or are some groups disproportionately benefiting after a recommendation while others lag behind (process and clinical outcome) (Davidson et al., 2021)?

Many questions are of course addressed and provisionally answered in the initial efficacy studies, but as these programs are promulgated, implemented, and disseminated over time, questions related to effectiveness should arise. A primary question is how a program's "real-world" outcomes compare to those of the initial trials. The outcomes may change because of training (practitioners in real-world settings may be trained and incentivized differently than those in a trial), and there may not be sufficient fiscal and skilled personnel resources available. This may lead to a program that is implemented differently than the program that was evaluated in the efficacy studies. In addition, underlying technologies and protocols may change, as may the target populations or the disease natural histories. All of these factors may influence the effectiveness of the disseminated program. AHRQ, working with relevant government agencies and key stakeholders, can develop programs to improve the evaluation of the effect of USPSTF CPGs.

COMMITTEE VISION

The committee developed a vision as to how the taxonomy and larger report recommendations would serve AHRQ's and ODP's goals to address evidence gaps in clinical prevention research. The vision encompasses activities, outputs, short-term outcomes, and long-term outcomes (see Figure S-3 and Chapter 5 for more detail). The committee approached the taxonomy and recommendations as an important component of a much larger effort for AHRQ, ODP, and USPSTF partners and other stakeholders to improve clinical prevention research and practice. They may find success in this endeavor not only by implementing this committee's taxonomy and recommendations but also by adapting the committee's vision to improve clinical prevention research and practice in the United States. The committee acknowledges that to do so will increase the burden on AHRQ and NIH staff and the USPSTF members. Resources will be needed to accomplish this.

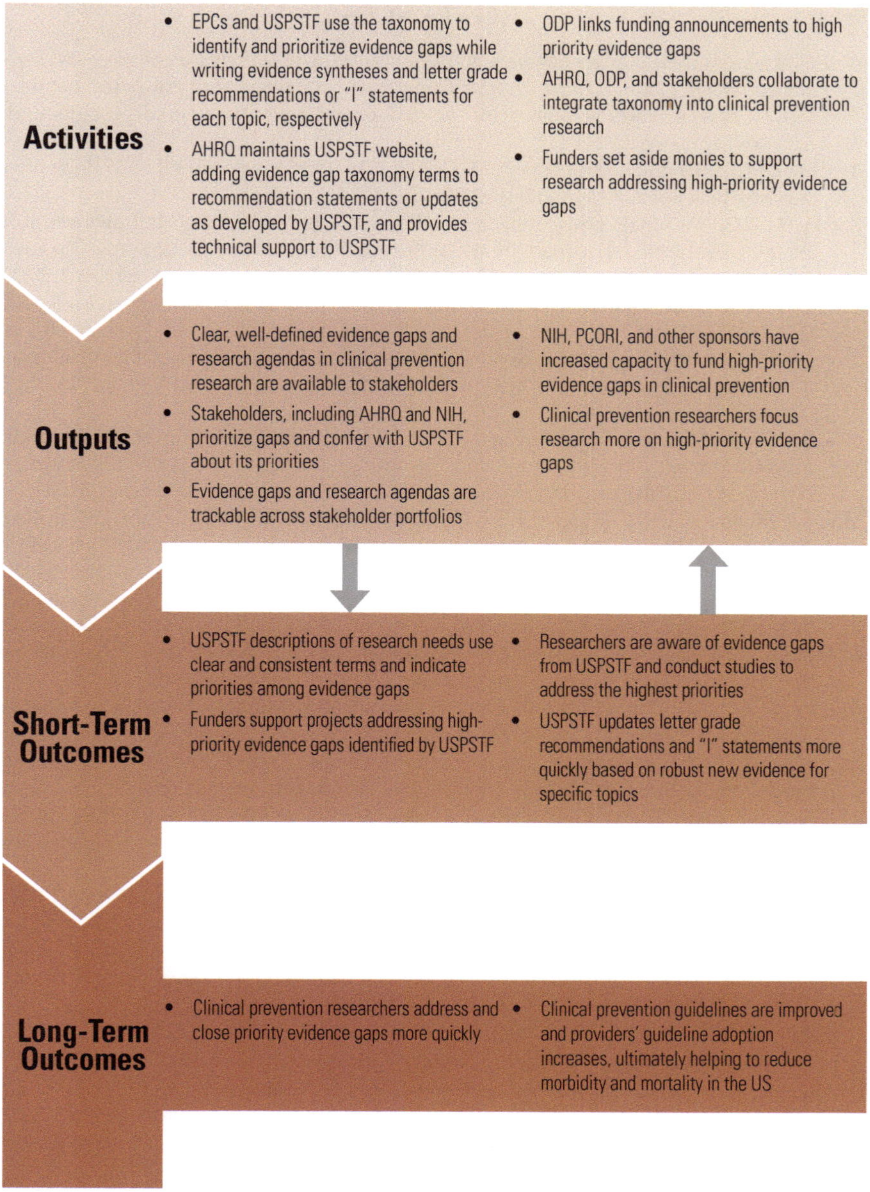

FIGURE S-3 The committee's vision for the report and taxonomy's role in improving clinical research by addressing evidence gaps.
NOTE: AHRQ = Agency for Healthcare Research and Quality; EPC = Evidence-based Practice Center; NIH = National Institutes of Health; ODP = Office of Disease Prevention; PCORI = Patient-Centered Outcomes Research Institute; USPSTF = U.S. Preventive Services Task Force.

REFERENCES

AHRQ (Agency for Healthcare Research and Quality). 2018. *U.S. Preventive Services Task Force procedures for Evidence-based Practice Centers.* https://www.ahrq.gov/sites/default/files/wysiwyg/funding/contracts/epc-vi/2-uspstf_procedures_guide_for_epcs.pdf (accessed November 3, 2021).

Bauchner, H., P. B. Fontanarosa, and R. M. Golub. 2016. JAMA welcomes the US Preventive Services Task Force. *JAMA* 315(4):351–352.

Borsky, A. 2021. Personal correspondence with Amanda Borsky, AHRQ staff member, July 29, 2021. Available by request from the project Public Access File at https://www8.nationalacademies.org/pa/ManageRequest.aspx?key=51932 (accessed November 3, 2021).

Davidson, K. W., A. H. Krist, C. Tseng, M. Simon, C. A. Doubeni, A. R. Kemper, M. Kubik, Q. Ngo-Metzger, J. Mills, and A. Borsky. 2021. Incorporation of social risk in US Preventive Services Task Force recommendations and identification of key challenges for primary care. *JAMA* 326(14):1410–1415. https://doi.org/10.1001/jama.2021.12833 (accessed October 19, 2021).

CTFPHE (Canadian Task Force on the Periodic Health Examination). 1979. The periodic health examination. *Canadian Medical Association Journal* 121(9):1193–1254. https://www.ncbi.nlm.nih.gov/pmc/articles/PMC1801737 (accessed November 2, 2021).

Mabry-Hernandez, I. R., S. J. Curry, W. R. Phillips, F. A. Garcia, K. W. Davidson, J. W. Epling, Jr., Q. Ngo-Metzger, and A. S. Bierman. 2018. US Preventive Services Task Force priorities for prevention research. *American Journal of Preventive Medicine* 54(1S1):S95–S103.

Mahase, E. 2021. US taskforce advises against low dose aspirin for primary prevention of cardiovascular disease. *BMJ* 375:n2521.

McGinnis, J. M., and S. H. Woolf. 1990. Background and objectives of the US Preventive Services Task Force. *Journal of General Internal Medicine* 5(5 Suppl):S11–S13.

Murray, D. M. 2017. Prevention research at the National Institutes of Health. *Public Health Reports* 132(5):535–538.

Murray, D. 2020. *Closing evidence gaps in clinical prevention: A perspective from the NIH.* Presented on December 15, 2020, at Meeting 1 of the Committee on Addressing Evidence Gaps in Clinical Prevention. https://www.nationalacademies.org/event/12-15-2020/addressing-evidence-gaps-in-clinical-prevention-committee-meeting-1-session-2 (accessed September 15, 2021).

NASEM (National Academies of Sciences, Engineering, and Medicine). 2020. *Meeting 1 (open session).* https://www.nationalacademies.org/event/12-15-2020/addressing-evidence-gaps-in-clinical-prevention-committee-meeting-1-session-2 (accessed September 15, 2021).

NIH (National Institutes of Health). 2020. *What we do: Budget.* https://www.nih.gov/about-nih/what-we-do/budget (accessed August 10, 2021).

Rabin, R. C. 2021. Aspirin use to prevent 1st heart attack or stroke should be curtailed, U.S. Panel says. *The New York Times.* https://www.nytimes.com/2021/10/12/health/aspirin-heart-attack-stroke.html (accessed November 3, 2021).

USPSTF (U.S. Preventive Services Task Force). 2017. *Update on methods: Insufficient evidence.* https://www.uspreventiveservicestaskforce.org/uspstf/about-uspstf/methods-and-processes/update-methods-insufficient-evidence (accessed July 19, 2021).

USPSTF. 2021a. *Aspirin use to prevent cardiovascular disease: Preventive medication.* https://www.uspreventiveservicestaskforce.org/uspstf/draft-recommendation/aspirin-use-to-prevent-cardiovascular-disease-preventive-medication (accessed October 27, 2021).

USPSTF. 2021b. *Procedure manual section 3: Topic workplan development.* https://www.uspreventiveservicestaskforce.org/uspstf/about-uspstf/methods-and-processes/procedure-manual/procedure-manual-section-3-topic-work-plan-development (accessed October 25, 2021).

USPSTF. 2021c. *USPSTF and cost considerations.* https://www.uspreventiveservicestaskforce.org/uspstf/about-uspstf/task-force-resources/uspstf-and-cost-considerations (accessed November 9, 2021).

USPSTF. n.d. *About the USPSTF.* https://www.uspreventiveservicestaskforce.org/uspstf/about-uspstf (accessed July 19, 2021).

1

Introduction

Clinical preventive services play an essential role in decreasing death and disability and improving the health of the nation. Preventive services such as breast cancer screenings, counseling on tobacco cessation, and preventive medication to decrease risk of HIV infection help to prevent certain diseases and, in some cases, enable early detection and treatment. The Patient Protection and Affordable Care Act (ACA), signed into law in 2010, required health plans to cover 100 percent of preventive services without charging patients for coinsurance, copayments, or deductibles. These services are identified as those that "provide coverage for a range of preventive services and may not impose cost-sharing" on patients receiving the services (KFF, 2015). Preventive services that are recommended by the U.S. Preventive Services Task Force (USPSTF), the Advisory Committee on Immunization Practices, the Health Resources and Services Administration (HRSA) (including HRSA's Bright Futures Project), and the Institute of Medicine's Committee on Women's Clinical Preventive Services are all required to be covered at no cost to patients (HRSA, 2020).

The USPSTF has issued clinical practice guidelines (CPGs) since 1989, recommending for or against clinical preventive services, including screenings, behavioral counseling, and preventive medication. In addition to providing recommendations for or against the use of specific interventions, the USPSTF highlights current gaps in the evidence base for a particular topic. They do so in recommendation statements as well as I statements, which are issued for preventive services about which there is insufficient evidence to issue a recommendation. The USPSTF have included evidence gaps since the first edition of its *Clinical Guide* was published. However, there have been limited efforts to systematize the identification of evidence gaps in prevention research, resulting in limited information about the impact such work has had on the research field as a whole. There is also limited evidence regarding the impact of the USPSTF's evidence gap identification in catalyzing prevention research agendas and studies that will enable a topic to be reviewed and updated. The purpose of this report is to (1) review the recommendation statements in the USPSTF portfolio and outline how evidence gaps are described; (2) suggest a taxonomy of evidence gaps and research needs for use in prevention research; (3) discuss novel research methodology that is needed to inform evidence gaps; and (4) propose new opportunities for collaboration among prevention researchers, funders, and guideline developers to accelerate prevention research that will close priority evidence gaps.

STATEMENT OF TASK

In an effort to close evidence gaps in clinical prevention, the Agency for Healthcare Research and Quality (AHRQ) and the National Institutes of Health's (NIH's) Office of Disease Prevention (ODP) contracted with the National Academies of Sciences, Engineering, and Medicine to convene an ad hoc committee to evaluate evidence gaps described by the USPSTF and other CPG developers and create a taxonomy of the evidence gaps that the USPSTF and other CPG developers could use in future recommendations. Furthermore, the committee was asked to provide methods for prevention research funders and recommendation statement developers, including but not limited to NIH and the USPSTF, to improve their partnerships to accelerate research to close important gaps in prevention (see Box 1-1 for the complete Statement of Task).

At the committee's first meeting, David Murray, director of ODP, characterized the challenges in addressing evidence gaps in two ways: nonspecific descriptions (e.g., "high-quality studies on the potential harms of screening and treatment are needed") and discussion of evidence gaps in various places (Murray, 2020). Expressly stated was the hope to link evidence gaps with USPSTF criteria for study inclusion and coordinated efforts to describe and communicate evidence gaps so that they are easier to identify and address (Murray, 2020).

Arlene Bierman, director of AHRQ's Center for Evidence and Practice Improvement, reinforced that the audience for the committee's work was threefold: recommendation-making bodies, research funders, and researchers. Bierman also emphasized that the taxonomy and recommendations should account for the multiple dimensions of evidence gaps

BOX 1-1
Statement of Task

An ad hoc committee of the National Academies of Sciences, Engineering, and Medicine will be convened to examine current issues in identifying and filling evidence gaps in U.S. Preventive Services Task Force (USPSTF) clinical prevention recommendations. As part of its work, the committee will:

- Catalog the evidence gaps identified in USPSTF recommendations.
- Develop a taxonomy of evidence gaps.
- Develop a summary of types of USPSTF evidence gaps to better communicate these gaps to funders and researchers.
- Identify potential research strategies that could help close specific types of identified evidence gaps.
- Suggest ways in which the National Institutes of Health and the Agency for Healthcare Research and Quality can enhance their partnership to optimize program announcements and requests for applications to accelerate research to close evidence gaps.

(Bierman, 2020). Furthermore, discussions with AHRQ staff supporting the USPSTF and the USPSTF chair indicated that other goals for the committee are to provide immediate and long-term solutions that will help:

- Organizations that develop preventive services recommendations, such as the USPSTF, to more clearly communicate evidence gaps;
- Funding agencies, including NIH, to understand, assess the relative importance of, and use evidence gaps from preventive services recommendations in order to ultimately support research to fill the gaps;
- Members of the research community to focus their research on high-priority areas that have evidence gaps; and
- All stakeholders, including patients, to accelerate the translation of evidence gaps into funding opportunities and other initiatives that ultimately use innovative methods to close evidence gaps related to clinical preventive services (Bierman, 2020).

These discussions led the committee to understand that their taxonomy and recommendations should not be constrained by the history and current practices of the USPSTF.

COMMITTEE PROCESS

The committee held four open sessions to solicit input on its statement of task, the experiences of others in developing taxonomies, and the challenges for NIH and researchers to address I statements. The committee reviewed literature on taxonomies and, in an iterative fashion, developed and modified a taxonomy using 12 I statements as test candidates for the taxonomy. The committee selected a number of I statements to use as exemplars in developing its taxonomy. Throughout the report, the committee focuses on two specific I statements: Screening for Cognitive Impairment in Older Adults and Screening with ECG for Atrial Fibrillation. The committee also developed a workflow to show how to use its taxonomy to develop a research agenda.

The committee emphasized the USPSTF's commitment to clinical prevention research as a means to advance health equity. The committee describes many opportunities that the USPSTF has to promote health equity in its work, starting with its topic identification and prioritization process. Where the committee saw an opportunity to advance health equity within this process, it has done so.

After identifying the long-term outcomes expected from the efforts led by AHRQ, ODP, and the USPSTF, the committee worked backward to assess what role its report (including the taxonomy) would play in AHRQ's and ODP's goals to improve clinical prevention research by addressing evidence gaps. The committee believes that the taxonomy and report's recommendations will play an important but singular part in this undertaking. Knowing that the long-term outcome is to identify and close evidence gaps in clinical prevention research (particularly those gaps informed by letter grade recommendations and I statements issued by the USPSTF) more quickly, the committee outlines the process it believes will ultimately lead AHRQ, ODP, and the USPSTF to this outcome in Figure 5-1 (see Chapter 5). The committee identifies the activities, outputs, and outcomes that are necessary to achieve this impact, including the use of the evidence gaps taxonomy and other recommendations made by the committee in this report. Because the vision incorporates activities and outputs defined in the recommendations in this report, the figure and full description can be found in Chapter 5.

Although the figure is neither strictly a logic model nor theory of change, it incorporates elements of both. The committee's vision includes the overall linearity of a logic model, articulating activities, outputs, and outcomes, and acknowledging that many elements within those categories already exist or have already been implemented by AHRQ, ODP, or the USPSTF. The vision also includes the assumptions and indicators associated with theories of change "through which the outcomes and activities work to achieve the desired impact" (Breuer et al., 2015; De Silva et al., 2014, p. 3).

ORGANIZATION OF THE REPORT

Chapter 2 describes the history and methods of the USPSTF, including how it and other CPG developers describe insufficient evidence. Chapter 3 describes the research enterprise involved in producing evidence for the USPSTF. Chapter 4 includes the taxonomy developed by the committee and describes how it can be used as part of a process to develop an actionable research agenda for USPSTF evidence gaps. Chapter 5 contains the committee's recommendations, which are focused on three areas: using the taxonomy, fostering clinical prevention research, and advancing the work of the USPSTF. The chapter also describes the committee's vision for improving clinical prevention research. Appendix A contains a comprehensive list of current I statements. Appendix B contains a description of research methods. Appendix C contains agendas from the committee's public meetings. Appendix D contains the committee members' and staff biographies. Appendix E contains summaries of the USPSTF's annual reports to Congress. Appendix F reviews the research needs identified by the USPSTF in select I Statements.

REFERENCES

Bierman, A. S. 2020. *Closing evidence gaps in clinical prevention: A perspective from AHRQ*. Presented on December 15, 2020, at Meeting 1 of the Committee on Addressing Evidence Gaps in Clinical Prevention. https://www.nationalacademies.org/event/12-15-2020/addressing-evidence-gaps-in-clinical-prevention-committee-meeting-1-session-2 (accessed October 22, 2021).

Breuer, E., L. Lee, M. De Silva, and C. Lund. 2015. Using theory of change to design and evaluate public health interventions: A systematic review. *Implementation Science* 11(63).

De Silva, M. J., E. Breuer, L. Lee, L. Asher, N. Chowdhary, C. Lund, and V. Patel. 2014. Theory of change: A theory-driven approach to enhance the Medical Research Council's framework for complex interventions. *Trials* 15(267). https://doi.org/10.1186/1745-6215-15-267 (accessed November 22, 2021).

HRSA (Health Resources and Services Administration). 2020. *Women's preventive services guidelines*. https://www.hrsa.gov/womens-guidelines-2019 (accessed July 19, 2021).

KFF (Kaiser Family Foundation). 2015. *Preventive services covered by private health plans under the Affordable Care Act*. https://www.kff.org/health-reform/fact-sheet/preventive-services-covered-by-private-health-plans (accessed July 19, 2021).

Murray, D. 2020. *Closing evidence gaps in clinical prevention: A perspective from the NIH*. Presented on December 15, 2020, at Meeting 1 of the Committee on Addressing Evidence Gaps in Clinical Prevention. https://www.nationalacademies.org/event/12-15-2020/addressing-evidence-gaps-in-clinical-prevention-committee-meeting-1-session-2 (accessed September 15, 2021).

2

Clinical Practice Guidelines and the U.S. Preventive Services Task Force

WHAT ARE CLINICAL PRACTICE GUIDELINES?

Since their proliferation in clinical settings in the United States in the late 1970s, clinical practice guidelines (CPGs) have evolved, and there is a preference for those that explicitly emphasize the use of the evidence base when possible (IOM, 2011; Weisz et al., 2007). In 2011, the Institute of Medicine defined CPGs as "statements that include recommendations intended to optimize patient care that are informed by a systematic review of evidence and an assessment of the benefits and harms of alternative care options" (IOM, 2011, p. 15). The systematic reviews that inform CPGs tend to reveal evidence gaps as well, though CPG developers have varying approaches to addressing them. Some CPG developers explicitly limit their statements to evidence-based recommendations, while others make recommendations in the absence of sufficient evidence using alternative approaches. The U.S. Preventive Services Task Force (USPSTF) and several other guideline developers prefer the former approach.

While the committee's statement of task included developing a taxonomy of evidence gaps and suggesting approaches to closing evidence gaps in clinical prevention in general, it explicitly named the USPSTF several times. For this reason, the committee approached the taxonomy as a tool for use beyond the Agency for Healthcare Research and Quality (AHRQ), the National Institutes of Health's (NIH's) Office of Disease Prevention (ODP), and the USPSTF, but kept the USPSTF in the main point of focus.

Barriers to Implementing Clinical Practice Guidelines

The USPSTF's scope is to "make recommendations on clinical preventive services to primary care clinicians," including screening tests, behavioral counseling, and preventive medications. The USPSTF recommendations *only* address services offered in primary care settings or those to which primary care clinicians can refer (USPSTF, n.d.-d). However, several contexts pose a threat to the broad dissemination and implementation of these recommendations, particularly in underserved or diverse clinical settings. There are many types of contextual barriers to implementing clinical guidelines, including but not limited to the health organization system and health professional context; guidelines context; patient context; and legal, social, and political contexts (Correa et al., 2020; Hurwitz, 1999). These barriers can also influence the equity of access to, use of, and receipt of health care.

Guidelines Context

Specific barriers to implementation in the guideline context may be simpler to resolve, but they include both lack of access or awareness of the existence of guidelines and an awareness of too many different guidelines regarding the same subject (Rauh et al., 2018). They also include beliefs regarding the credibility of the evidence base (or lack thereof), or that the recommendation is impractical to implement (Correa et al., 2020). Another guideline-related barrier includes the belief that guidelines "restrict clinical judgment, challenge professional autonomy, and limit treatment options" (Correa et al., 2020, p. 6).

Health Professional and Health Systems Context(s)

Barriers in the health professional context center on clinician attitudes and behaviors having to do with their own autonomy, their practice, their patients, or all three. Clinicians may be unable to implement or may actively avoid implementing for a variety of reasons. These include variations in priorities between clinicians and the health systems in which they work; clinicians having more confidence in their own clinical experience than in guidelines; clinician resistance to change or doubts about the efficacy of an intervention, or perceived loss of autonomy in following guidelines; or a lack of communication between clinicians regarding best practices for implementation (Correa et al., 2020).

Health systems also face barriers to implementing CPGs. Health systems may struggle with a lack of clear protocols or processes to successfully implement new guidelines, and they may lack tools or resources to provide certain services. They may also lack services in their communities to which they would refer patients (e.g., psychiatric care to which a patient could be referred after being screened for depression) (Anthony et al., 2010). New guidelines can be challenging to implement when the recommendation reduces the frequency of a current standard practice, particularly when both clinicians and patients are accustomed to the current practice. Reductions in services in particular may concern health systems that implementation will result in reduced patient visits and thus revenue (Fischer et al., 2016; IOM, 2011). Health systems may also lack resources and equipment to implement certain recommendations.

Clinicians and health systems may also feel they are too busy or overwhelmed with their current caseloads and be disinclined to incorporate additional services into their work (Fischer et al., 2016). Priorities for specific health conditions or services may also vary by health system or provider, leading to different services being offered (Harding et al., 2014).

Patient Context

The patient context is another consideration when implementing CPGs. Patients may be reluctant to request or accept suggestions for a service for a variety of reasons, including limited language, literacy, or health literacy; limited motivation to follow a certain recommendation; or concerns about affordability. They may also turn down offers of preventive services based on fears of real or perceived harms (Jones et al., 2010). Conversely, they may request a preventive service more frequently than is recommended, particularly if the suggested frequency of a service is reduced in a new recommendation statement (Allen et al., 2013). Patients may be suspicious that a reduction in frequency is a "cost-savings measure by insurers and/or providers" (Allen et al., 2013, p. 1).

Legal and Sociopolitical Context(s)

Legal and sociopolitical contexts may relate specifically to a health system organization's or other practice's work culture and are described above. Additional legal and sociopolitical contexts include case law related to CPGs. Some courts have upheld CPGs as national legal standards for care, while others have disregarded them in favor of local standards for care (Merenstein, 2004). This uncertainty can lead to clinicians ordering more diagnostic tests for patients than is recommended, for fear of malpractice lawsuits (IOM, 2011).

Barriers to implementing CPGs can also reflect and reinforce health disparities (Welch et al., 2017). Guideline-issuing bodies do not always consider equity when developing recommendations, possibly contributing to additional difficulties implementing them in underserved or marginalized communities (Lang et al., 2021). As mentioned earlier, the Patient Protection and Affordable Care Act of 2010 (ACA) requires private health insurers to provide certain preventive services at no cost to patients (KFF, 2015). However, despite this provision, patients with employer-covered insurance are still paying between $75 million and $219 million annually for preventive care, according to a recent estimate by Hoagland and Shafer (2021).

U.S. PREVENTIVE SERVICES TASK FORCE

History and Scope

In 1984, the U.S. Department of Health and Human Services (HHS) assistant secretary Edward N. Brandt commissioned the USPSTF to "improve the health of people nationwide by making evidence-based recommendations about clinical preventive services" (USPSTF, 2021a). The USPSTF was assembled as an effort to continue and expand the innovative work of the Canadian Task Force on the Periodic Health Examination (CTFPHE), which was founded in 1976 and began issuing preventive service recommendations in the late 1970s (CTFPHE, 1979; McGinnis and Woolf, 1990). The CTFPHE's report laid out the basic elements of preventive evidence assessment as they lead to clinical recommendations. These included comprehensively reviewing the literature; prioritizing methods for assessing individual interventions, including determining the burden of suffering and ability to measure outcomes; understanding the risks and benefits of an intervention; rating the effectiveness of interventions; grading the level of evidence for a recommendation; and defining a research agenda to address unanswered questions (CTFPHE, 1979). As an independent, volunteer panel of 20 experts in clinical prevention and evidence-based medicine,[1] the USPSTF sought to examine "more current issues in preventive medicine and more recent evidence not available to [the CTFPHE] and to move the debate forward into new areas not previously addressed" (McGinnis and Woolf, 1990, p. S12). Its objectives were to develop risk factor–specific recommendations for CPGs, address behavioral and structural barriers to prevention, and develop a prevention research agenda (McGinnis and Woolf, 1990).

Because the USPSTF adopted the methodology used by the CTFPHE, the two bodies were able to collaborate "in a binational effort to review evidence and develop recommendations on preventive services," (USPSTF, 1989) sending and receiving members to each other's meetings (McGinnis and Woolf, 1990). In 1989, the USPSTF published its first report on CPGs, *Guide to Clinical Preventive Services: An Assessment of the Effectiveness of 169 Interventions*, and was disbanded (USPSTF, 1989).

---

[1] The USPSTF currently comprises 16 members each serving 4-year terms.

The second task force was assembled in September 1990 and met through April 1994 (USPSTF, 1996). The task force received support from HHS's Office of Disease Prevention and Health Promotion and Agency for Healthcare Policy and Research (AHCPR) to "analyze systematically scientific evidence pertaining to clinical preventive services that had been published since the first edition of the *Guide*" (USPSTF, 1996, p. xxix). In 1999, the U.S. Congress reauthorized AHCPR and renamed it the Agency for Healthcare Research and Quality (AHRQ). The legislation also states that the USPSTF

> shall review the scientific evidence related to the effectiveness, appropriateness, and cost-effectiveness of clinical preventive services for the purpose of developing recommendations for the health care community, and updating previous clinical preventive recommendations.[2]

However, despite having the authority to do so, the USPSTF does not evaluate evidence related to cost-effectiveness when issuing a grade for a topic:

> [USPSTF] excludes costs from its determination of the benefits and harms of a clinical preventive service. This deliberate decision was made to maintain a clear focus on the science of clinical effectiveness (i.e., "what works"), and not consider cost, in part to avoid any misperception that the Task Force's purpose is to limit health care based on cost.... The Task Force recognizes that cost is a consideration for insurers, health systems, purchasers, and consumers. The USPSTF maintains that regardless of how health care is financed, it is essential to understand what the science says about which preventive services work. (USPSTF, 2021c)

Congress also authorized the AHRQ director to convene and appoint members to the USPSTF, and authorized AHRQ to "provide ongoing administrative, research, and technical support for [USPSTF] operations, including coordinating and supporting the dissemination of [its] recommendations."[3] AHRQ published the third and final edition of the original *Guide* in 2002 (USPSTF, 2002). By 2005, AHRQ had been publishing the USPSTF's recommendations as they were issued for each topic online, as well as "pocket guides" with abridged recommendations the

---

[2] 106th U.S. Congress, First Session. Public Law 106-129, Section 915. Healthcare Research and Quality Act of 1999. https://www.ahrq.gov/sites/default/files/wysiwyg/policymakers/hrqa99.pdf (accessed July 20, 2021).

[3] 106th U.S. Congress, First Session. Public Law 106-129, Section 915. Healthcare Research and Quality Act of 1999. https://www.ahrq.gov/sites/default/files/wysiwyg/policymakers/hrqa99.pdf (accessed July 20, 2021).

task force had issued individually in the preceding years (USPSTF, 2005, 2007a, 2009, 2010, 2012, 2014a).

U.S. Preventive Services Task Force Process

The process of selecting a topic for review through publishing the final recommendation statement takes 3 years on average (Borsky, 2021). Presently, the USPSTF process for reviewing and developing recommendations begins with soliciting topics for nomination (USPSTF, 2021d) (see Figure 2-1). Any individual or organization can nominate a topic at any time; the USPSTF identifies those that are within its scope and prioritizes each one with the input of its stakeholders and partner liaisons. The task force then works with one of the Evidence-based Practice Centers (EPCs) supported by AHRQ to develop a draft research plan, which is posted for public comment. After the USPSTF and the EPC review and

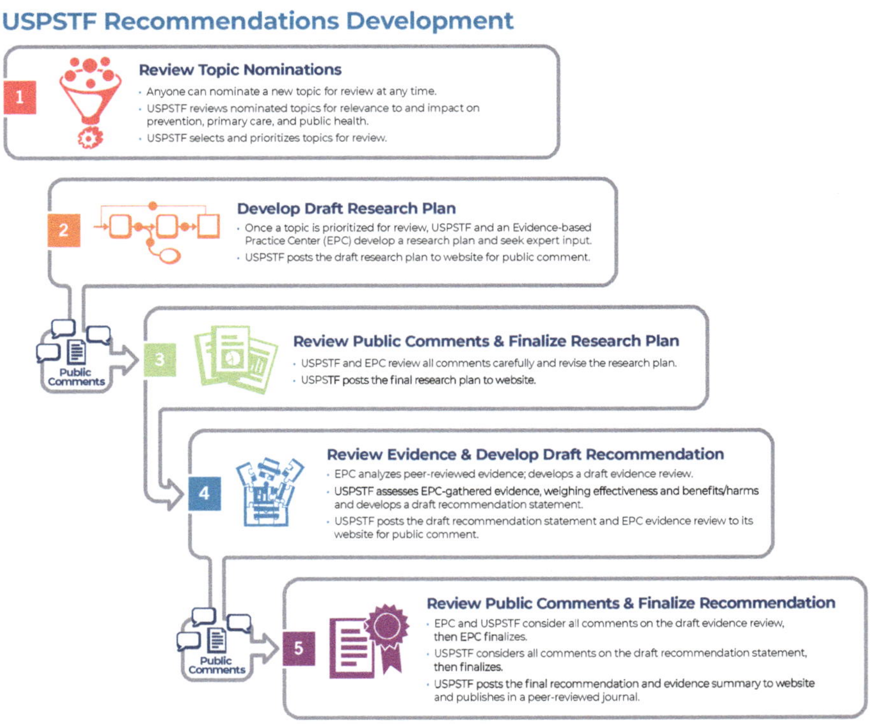

FIGURE 2-1 U.S. Preventive Services Task Force recommendations development process: a graphic overview.
SOURCE: USPSTF, 2021d.

revise as needed, the final plan is posted online. The EPC conducts the systematic review according to the research plan, and the USPSTF begins assessing the evidence after the EPC sends its draft review. The USPSTF then drafts a recommendation statement and posts it online for public comment, and after a review of public comments the EPC finalizes its evidence review. The USPSTF then finalizes its recommendation statement, and both are posted online, and as of 2016, published in a journal of the JAMA Network (Bauchner et al., 2016). The USPSTF also considers previously graded topics for updates starting 2–3 years after they are first published, first soliciting stakeholder input and examining the likelihood that enough new evidence has been developed that the recommendation for practice may be updated.

The development of recommendations for preventive services "typically requires deliberation using comprehensive systematic reviews of the best available evidence and a series of complex judgments" (USPSTF, 2019). The USPSTF assessment of the overall evidence for a clinical preventive service requires two key determinations: "assessment of the degree of certainty about the net benefit (benefits minus harms) and assessment of the magnitude of net benefit for the population for whom the service is intended" (for a visual of this matrix, see Table 2-1) (USPSTF, 2019).

Grading Scheme

The USPSTF last updated its methods for understanding certainty and net benefit and linking intermediate outcomes and health outcomes in prevention in 2018 (USPSTF, 2018). The USPSTF updated its grading scheme most recently in 2012 and prior to that in 2007 (USPSTF, 2018). Currently, grades A and B indicate that the task force recommends an intervention, grade C indicates selectively offering a service, and grade D indicates that the task force recommends against implementing a pre-

TABLE 2-1 Matrix of Assessing Certainty and Magnitude of Net Benefit Used by the U.S. Preventive Services Task Force

Certainty of Net Benefit	Magnitude of Net Benefit			
	Substantial	Moderate	Small	Zero/Negative
High	A	B	C	D
Moderate	B	B	C	D
Low	Insufficient (I Statement)			

ventive service. The task force makes these assessments by evaluating the evidence using the following steps:

1. Assessing the adequacy of evidence at the key question level.
2. Assessing the adequacy of evidence at the linkage level.
3. Estimating the magnitude of benefit and harm of the preventive service.
4. Evaluating the certainty of the evidence for net benefit for the preventive service.
5. Estimating the magnitude of the net benefit of the preventive service.
6. Developing a recommendation grade for the preventive service in the relevant population, based on the above parameters (USPSTF, 2017a).

Evidence Gaps and I Statements

While the recommendations for or against a clinical service receive a grade, some topics are given I statements, indicating that the USPSTF has not found sufficient evidence to make a recommendation at all. In 2009, the task force announced that it would shift from using the phrase "I recommendation" to "I statement" to reduce confusion among clinicians about whether a topic with an I was recommended or not (USPSTF, 2017b). Topics can receive an I statement instead of a graded recommendation due to lack of evidence, a lack of good quality evidence, or an abundance of conflicting evidence. Without clear or good quality evidence, the USPSTF cannot determine the balance of benefits and harms and does not make a recommendation about the provision of the service. As of the publication of this report, 53 topics have I statements either for a specific subpopulation or for recommending the service at all (see Appendix A). On average, 8.4 years elapse before a preventive service with an I statement is issued a definitive grade recommendation by the USPSTF, if it is to receive one at all (Klabunde et al., 2021).

While I statement text is usually centered around identifying the missing evidence that must be developed in order to update a topic with a letter grade, recommendations with letter grades also identify evidence gaps and research needs either to reinforce or change recommendations or to generally advance prevention research on the topic. Since 1989, USPSTF recommendations have suggested evidence gaps or research needs for various topics in one way or another, but in 2007, the USPSTF introduced a new section of its recommendation statements called "Other Considerations." This section could include cost and dissemination and implementation considerations for clinicians and policymakers, as well as "key gaps in the evidence and ... priorities for future research and research funding" (Barton et al., 2007, p. 125). In 2019, however, another methods update restructured the section to give "Research Needs and Gaps" its own section. The details of those sections vary widely in specificity and scope. See Appendix F.

A small number of the USPSTF's 129 recommendations are currently marked as "archived," "inactive," or "referred" and refer users to other guideline developers. Two refer users to the Advisory Committee on Immunization Practice (for information on adult and child immunization practices) (USPSTF, n.d.-a, n.d.-b), and two refer users to the Discretionary Advisory Committee on Heritable Disorders in Newborns and Children (for information related to phenylketonuria and sickle cell disease screenings) (USPSTF, 2008, n.d.-c). The other two refer users to the Community Guide website (for information related to using seatbelts and preventing motor vehicle injury, and preventing youth violence) (USPSTF, 2007b, 2014b).

This committee was charged with the task of developing a taxonomy to characterize types of evidence gaps and research needs in clinical prevention research, particularly as they relate to topics considered by the USPSTF. When reviewing a preventive service, the USPSTF may find there is insufficient evidence to assess whether the service (or certain individuals potentially receiving a preventive service) should be recommended for a variety of reasons. For example, insufficient evidence may relate to limited effectiveness of interventions; questionable value of early intervention; conflicting evidence of existing studies; limited treatment evidence in lower-risk subgroups; subclinical vs clinical endpoints; and variable impact of screen-detected disease (Atkins, 2021). For examples of each, see Table 2-2.

New evidence reviewed to update a topic with an I statement may also not be enough to upgrade it to receive a letter grade recommendation. The ACA requires the USPSTF and the Community Preventive Services Task Force (CPSTF) to provide annual reports to Congress, outlining major evidence gaps in clinical prevention research and highlighting high-priority areas or topics that "deserve further examination" (USPSTF, 2020). Appendix E contains a list of all reports to Congress. Some research priority topics in recent years identified by the USPSTF have included adolescent health and health inequities, substance use, violence prevention, cancer prevention, and cardiovascular health. Since the USPSTF submitted its first annual report to Congress, some topics that originally had I statements no longer do, while others have had two or three updates with no change. For example, new evidence upgraded a recommendation

TABLE 2-2 Types of Evidence Gaps That May Lead to an I Statement for a Topic

Type of Gap	Example
Limited effectiveness of interventions	Tobacco cessation in teens Cognitive impairment in older adults (or age bracket) Suicide screening
Questionable value of earlier intervention	Vision screening in older adults
Conflicting evidence of existing studies	Calcium/vitamin D for fracture prevention
Limited treatment evidence in lower risk subgroups	AAA screening in women Osteoporosis in men
Subclinical versus clinical endpoints	Glaucoma treatment Osteoporosis treatment in men
Variable impact of screen-detected disease	Thyroid dysfunction Iron-deficiency

NOTE: AAA = abdominal aortic aneurysm.
SOURCES: Adapted from a presentation by David Atkins on March 16, 2021; Atkins, 2021.

around hearing loss in newborns from an I in 2001 to a B in 2008.[4] Additionally, the recommendation that clinicians screen children for obesity and offer or refer them to comprehensive, intensive behavioral intervention to promote improvement in weight status received an I statement in 2004 and was upgraded to a B in 2010, due to a "number of new studies" (USPSTF, 2011). In contrast, some I statements no longer exist because new evidence has changed the key questions about the preventive service itself. For example, in 2008, computed tomographic colonography and fecal DNA testing were a type of screening for colorectal cancer given an I statement by the USPSTF. When the USPSTF updated the colorectal cancer screening in 2016, new evidence about the harms and benefits of those screenings had already emerged, and the USPSTF updated its recommendation so that it no longer included an I statement or separate grade for those specific screenings. Computed tomographic colonography and fecal DNA testing were included in a list of other screenings that were recommended for certain age groups (regarding screening for colorectal cancer, adults aged 50–75 years received an A grade recommendation; adults aged 45–49 years received a B grade recommendation; and adults aged 76–86 years received a C grade recommendation).

Revisiting I statements, however, can engender substantial costs in time and fiscal resources, often without important yields in improved

[4] This recommendation has since been archived.

guidelines that will ultimately elevate community health status levels. There is also the problem of opportunity costs for selected USPSTF activities, as there may be nascent but promising interventions appearing that require attention. In addition, evidence gaps in I statements that are not well described can result in resources (time and money) squandered on research that will not help turn the I statement into a letter grade recommendation.

U.S. Preventive Services Task Force's Relationship with the Community Preventive Services Task Force

HHS established the CPSTF in 1996 to provide findings and recommendations about community preventive services, programs, and other interventions aimed at improving population health, and to complement the work of the USPSTF (CPSTF, n.d.-a). The collection of recommendations and findings made by the CPSTF are referred to as the *Community Guide*. As AHRQ supports the USPSTF, the Centers for Disease Control and Prevention (CDC) provides scientific and administrative support to the CPSTF. AHRQ and CDC staff members who support their respective task forces typically serve as partner liaisons for the other task force, attending the other's meetings regularly and occasionally presenting their relevant work. Many of the CPSTF organizational and methodological characteristics derive directly from those of the USPSTF (Briss et al., 2000; Truman et al., 2000). The CPSTF is also guided by the Healthy People Initiative, which identifies population targets for improved public health outcomes in advance of each decade (NASEM, 2020).

The USPSTF and the CPSTF both collaborate with ODP to communicate with NIH's institutes and centers (ICs) regarding evidence gaps and research needs identified in their evidence assessments. ODP disseminates newer I statements or insufficient evidence statements that have been issued by the task forces and collects information from the ICs about the relevant research they have funded (ODP, 2021). The CPSTF methodology contrasts with that of the USPSTF by focusing on interventions at the population level as opposed to the individual level, and thus more frequently evaluating a body of evidence in which "non-randomized studies commonly have behavioral outcomes as endpoints" (Grossman and Elder, 2015, p. 3). However, the more interactive complementary nature of the two task forces allows for the interventions recommended by the CPSTF to support the implementation and delivery of interventions recommended by the USPSTF. For example, the USPSTF recommends screening for colon and rectal cancer among adults aged 45–75 years, and the CPSTF recommends a multitude of different interventions to *increase* certain types of colon and rectal cancer screenings, including using reminder and recall systems, engaging community health workers, and reducing structural barriers for clients (CPSTF, 2005, 2006, 2009, 2010a,b,c, 2016, 2019; USPSTF, 2021b). The USPSTF's and the CPSTF's complementary work is visualized in Figure 2-2.

Like its methodology, the CPSTF's grades for findings differ from those of the USPSTF. The CPSTF will recommend for or against an intervention, and the strength of evidence is rated as "strong" or "sufficient." A crucial difference is that the USPSTF grades connote varying degrees of the magnitude of net benefit and the degree of certainty about it, while the CPSTF findings category of "strong" or "sufficient" is a direct evaluation of the quality of the evidence base and not a reflection of the expected magnitude of benefits (CPSTF, n.d.-c). The CPSTF may also find that an intervention has IE. An intervention may be given an IE grade if there is a lack of research available or inconsistent results that prevent the CPSTF from determining if an intervention should be recommended at all. The CPSTF has turned each IE finding into factsheets that are publicly available on its website for use by public health practitioners, researchers, and funders (CPSTF, n.d.-b). When describing evidence gaps in recommended topics, the CPSTF refers users specifically to the systematic review that

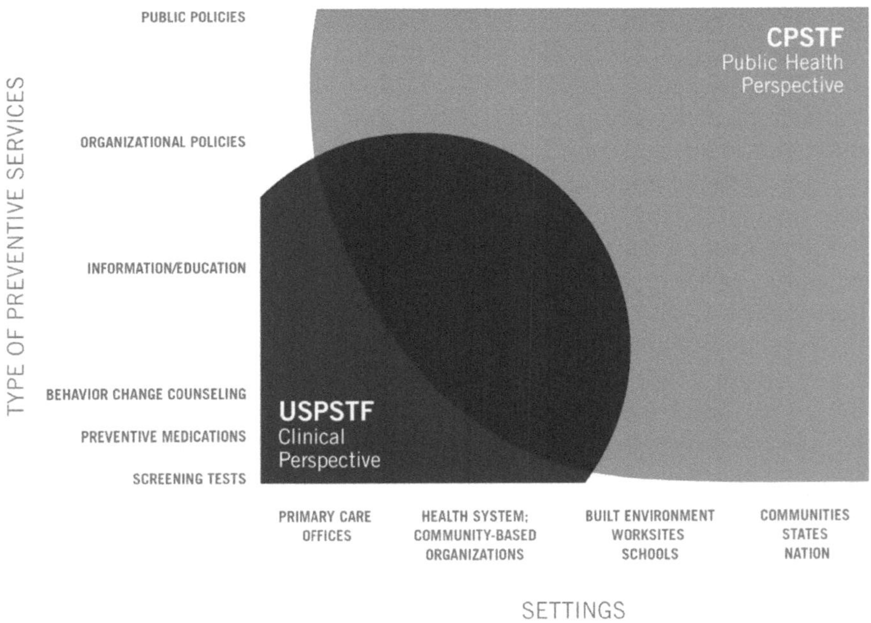

FIGURE 2-2 The relationship between the U.S. Preventive Services Task Force and the Community Preventive Services Task Force.
SOURCE: Grossman and Elder, 2015.

informed its assessment, and often uses the subcategories of "effectiveness," "applicability," and "implementation" to characterize evidence gaps.

HOW OTHER CLINICAL PRACTICE GUIDELINE DEVELOPERS ADDRESS EVIDENCE GAPS

The committee looked for possible helpful taxonomies from other CPG developers. While no such taxonomy was discovered, the search provided some insights into how other panels address insufficient evidence. For example, the American College of Cardiology and the American Heart Association and the United Kingdom National Screening Committee describe evidence gaps in a manner similar to those of the USPSTF's I statements or the CPSTSF's IEs, though nomenclature varies. If there is insufficient evidence regarding a service, they so state and do not recommend for or against the preventive service (Duff et al., 2019; Hamid et al., 2021).

Other bodies treat insufficient evidence differently. Instead of declining to recommend for or against a preventive service, some bodies use expert opinion to take the place of evidence when sufficient evidence is not available. With breast cancer screening, for example, the USPSTF issued a C grade for biennial mammograms in women aged 40–49 years, with moderate certainty that the net benefit of screening with mammography in women ages 40 through 49 is small (USPSTF, 2016). The American Cancer Society and the American College of Obstetricians and Gynecologists recommend breast cancer screening even for ages where it notes there are gaps in the evidence, based "primarily on consensus and expert opinion" (ACOG CPBG, 2017; Oeffinger et al., 2015).

Some groups produce disease-based guidelines (i.e., guidelines that discuss both prevention and treatment). As such, the noted research gaps span the prevention and treatment domains. Of note, some disease-based organizations assume the need to screen, so the research gaps do not always address the lack of demonstrated screening efficacy. For example, the Society for Vascular Surgery (SVS) provides a lengthy list of research gaps ("Areas in Need of Further Research") for abdominal aortic aneurysm (AAA), but these dealt more with improving processes of care than whether the screening for AAA should be done (Chaikof et al., 2009). Because practicing clinicians often need guidance, especially when there is insufficient evidence, the purpose of the following examples is to show the variety of responses to insufficient evidence, rather than to criticize particular guidelines for differing in methodology from the USPSTF.

REFERENCES

ACOG CPBG (American College of Obstetricians and Gynecologists Committee on Practice Bulletins—Gynecology). 2017. Breast cancer risk assessment and screening in average-risk women. *ACOG Practice Bulletin* 179. https://www.acog.org/clinical/clinical-guidance/practice-bulletin/articles/2017/07/breast-cancer-risk-assessment-and-screening-in-average-risk-women (accessed October 19, 2021).

Allen, J. D., S. M. Bluethmann, M. Sheets, K. M. Opdyke, K. Gates-Ferris, M. Hurlbert, and E. Harden. 2013. Women's responses to changes in U.S. Preventive Task Force's mammography screening guidelines: Results of focus groups with ethnically diverse women. *BMC Public Health* 13:1169. https://doi.org/10.1186/1471-2458-13-1169 (accessed October 19, 2021).

Anthony, J. S., S.-Y. Baik, B. J. Bowers, B. Tidjani, C. J. Jacobson, and J. Susman. 2010. Conditions that influence a primary care clinician's decision to refer patients for depression care. *Rehabilitation Nursing* 35(3):113–122. https://doi.org/10.1002/j.2048-7940.2010.tb00286.x (accessed November 2, 2021).

Atkins, D. 2021. *Funder perspectives on addressing evidence gaps*. Presented on March 16, 2021, at Meeting 4 of the Committee on Addressing Evidence Gaps in Clinical Prevention. https://www.nationalacademies.org/event/03-16-2021/addressing-evidence-gaps-in-clinical-prevention-committee-meeting-session-2 (accessed October 19, 2021).

Barton, M. B., T. Miller, T. Wolff, D. Petitti, M. LeFevre, G. Sawaya, B. Yawn, J. Guirguis-Blake, N. Calonge, R. Harris, and U.S. Preventive Services Task Force. 2007. How to read the new recommendation statement: Methods update from the U.S. Preventive Services Task Force. *Annals of Internal Medicine* 147(2):123–127. https://doi.org/10.7326/0003-4819-147-2-200707170-00171 (accessed October 19, 2021).

Bauchner, H., P. B. Fontanarosa, and R. M. Golub. 2016. JAMA welcomes the U.S. Preventive Services Task Force. *JAMA* 315(4):351–352. https://doi.org/10.1001/jama.2015.18448 (accessed October 19, 2021).

Borsky, A. 2021. Personal correspondence with Amanda Borsky, AHRQ staff member, July 29, 2021. Available by request from the project Public Access File at https://www8.nationalacademies.org/pa/ManageRequest.aspx?key=51932 (accessed November 3, 2021).

Briss, P. A., S. Zaza, M. Pappaioanou, J. Fielding, L. Wright-De Agüero, B. I. Truman, D. P. Hopkins, P. D. Mullen, R. S. Thompson, S. H. Woolf, V. G. Carande-Kulis, L. Anderson, A. R. Hinman, D. V. McQueen, S. M. Teutsch, and J. R. Harris. 2000. Developing an evidence-based guide to community preventive services—methods. The Task Force on Community Preventive Services. *American Journal of Preventive Medicine* 18(1 Suppl):35–43. https://doi.org/10.1016/S0749-3797(99)00119-1 (accessed October 19, 2021).

Chaikof, E. L., D. C. Brewster, R. L. Dalman, M. S. Makaroun, K. A. Illig, G. A. Sicard, C. H. Timaran, G. R. Upchurch, Jr., and F. J. Veith. 2009. The care of patients with an abdominal aortic aneurysm: The Society for Vascular Surgery practice guidelines. *Journal of Vascular Surgery* 50(4 Suppl):S2–S49. https://doi.org/10.1016/j.jvs.2017.10.044 (accessed October 19, 2021).

Correa, V. C., L. H. Lugo-Agudelo, D. C. Aguirre-Acevedo, J. A. P. Contreras, A. M. P. Borrero, D. F. Patino-Lugo, and D. A. C. Valencia. 2020. Individual, health system, and contextual barriers and facilitators for the implementation of clinical practice guidelines: A systematic metareview. *Health Research Policy and Systems* 18(1):74. https://health-policy-systems.biomedcentral.com/articles/10.1186/s12961-020-00588-8 (accessed October 19, 2021).

CPSTF (Community Preventive Services Task Force). 2005. *Cancer screening: Small media targeting clients—colorectal cancer.* https://www.thecommunityguide.org/findings/cancer-screening-small-media-targeting-clients-colorectal-cancer (accessed July 19, 2021).

CPSTF. 2006. *Cancer screening: Provider reminder and recall systems—colorectal cancer.* https://www.thecommunityguide.org/findings/cancer-screening-provider-reminder-and-recall-systems-colorectal-cancer (accessed July 19, 2021).

CPSTF. 2009. *Cancer screening: Provider assessment and feedback—colorectal cancer.* https://www.thecommunityguide.org/findings/cancer-screening-provider-assessment-and-feedback-colorectal-cancer (accessed July 19, 2021).

CPSTF. 2010a. *Cancer screening: Client reminders—colorectal cancer.* https://www.thecommunityguide.org/findings/cancer-screening-client-reminders-colorectal-cancer (accessed July 19, 2021).

CPSTF. 2010b. *Cancer screening: One-on-one education for clients—colorectal cancer.* https://www.thecommunityguide.org/findings/cancer-screening-one-one-education-clients-colorectal-cancer (accessed July 19, 2021).

CPSTF. 2010c. *Cancer screening: Reducing structural barriers for clients—colorectal cancer.* https://www.thecommunityguide.org/findings/cancer-screening-reducing-structural-barriers-clients-colorectal-cancer (accessed July 19, 2021).

CPSTF. 2016. *Cancer screening: Multicomponent interventions—colorectal cancer.* https://www.thecommunityguide.org/findings/cancer-screening-multicomponent-interventions-colorectal-cancer (accessed July 19, 2021).

CPSTF. 2019. *Cancer screening: Interventions engaging community health workers—colorectal cancer.* https://www.thecommunityguide.org/findings/cancer-screening-interventions-engaging-community-health-workers-colorectal-cancer (accessed July 19, 2021).

CPSTF. n.d.-a. *About the Community Preventive Services Task Force.* https://www.thecommunityguide.org/task-force/about-community-preventive-services-task-force (accessed July 19, 2021).

CPSTF. n.d.-b. *New resource outlines ways to use insufficient evidence findings.* https://www.thecommunityguide.org/content/new-resource-outlines-ways-use-insufficient-evidence-findings (accessed July 19, 2021).

CPSTF. n.d.-c. *Community Guide methodology.* https://www.thecommunityguide.org/about/community-guide-methodology (accessed July 19, 2021).

CTFPHE (Canadian Task Force on the Public Health Examination). 1979. The periodic health examination. *Canadian Medical Association Journal* 121(9):1193–1254. https://www.ncbi.nlm.nih.gov/pmc/articles/PMC1801737/ (accessed November 2, 2021).

Duff, J. P., A. A. Topjian, M. D. Berg, M. Chan, S. E. Haskell, B. L. Joyner, Jr., J. J. Lasa, S. J. Ley, T. T. Raymond, R. M. Sutton, M. F. Hazinski, and D. L. Atkins. 2019. 2019 American Heart Association focused update on pediatric advanced life support: An update to the American Heart Association guidelines for cardiopulmonary resuscitation and emergency cardiovascular care. *Circulation* 140:e904–e914. https://www.ahajournals.org/doi/10.1161/CIR.0000000000000731 (accessed October 19, 2021).

Fischer, F., K. Lange, K. Klose, W. Greiner, and A. Kraemer. 2016. Barriers and strategies in guideline implementation—a scoping review. *Healthcare (Basel)* 4(3):36.

Grossman, D. C., and R. W. Elder. 2015. Aligning the work of two U.S. task forces on behavioral counseling recommendations. *American Journal of Preventive Medicine* 49(3 Suppl 2):S174–S183.

Hamid, S., P. Desai, P. Hysi, J. M. Burr, and A. P. Khawaja. 2021. Population screening for glaucoma in UK: Current recommendations and future directions. *Eye.* https://doi.org/10.1038/s41433-021-01687-8 (accessed October 19, 2021).

Harding, K., J. Porter, A. Horne-Thompson, E. Donley, and N. F. Taylor. 2014. Not enough time or a low priority? Barriers to evidence-based practice for allied health clinicians. *Journal of Continuing Education in the Health Professions* 34(4):224–231.

Hoagland, A., and P. Shafer. 2021. Out-of-pocket costs for preventive care persist almost a decade after the Affordable Care Act. *Preventive Medicine* 150:106690.

Hurwitz, B. 1999. Legal and political considerations of clinical practice guidelines. *BMJ* 318(7184):661–664.

IOM (Institute of Medicine). 2011. *Clinical practice guidelines we can trust*. Washington, DC: The National Academies Press. https://doi.org/10.17226/13058.

Jones, R. M., K. J. Devers, A. J. Kuzel, and S. H. Woolf. 2010. Patient-reported barriers to colorectal cancer screening: A mixed-methods analysis. *American Journal of Preventive Medicine* 38(5):508–516.

KFF (Kaiser Family Foundation). 2015. *Preventive services covered by private health plans under the Affordable Care Act*. https://www.kff.org/health-reform/fact-sheet/preventive-services-covered-by-private-health-plans (accessed July 19, 2021).

Klabunde, C. N., E. M. Ellis, J. Villani, E. Neilson, K. Schwartz, E. A. Vogt, and Q. Ngo-Metzger. 2021. Characteristics of scientific evidence informing changed U.S. Preventive Services Task Force insufficient evidence statements. *American Journal of Preventive Medicine*. https://www.sciencedirect.com/science/article/abs/pii/S0749379721004578 (accessed November 29, 2021).

Lang, E., S. Alves da Silva, and N. Persaud. 2021. Are guidelines fueling inequity? A call to action for guideline developers and their panelists. *Chest* 159(2):465–466.

McGinnis, J. M., and S. H. Woolf. 1990. Background and objectives of the U.S. Preventive Services Task Force. *Journal of General Internal Medicine* 5(5 Suppl):S11–S13.

Merenstein, D. 2004. A piece of my mind. Winners and losers. *JAMA* 291(1):15–16.

NASEM (National Academies of Sciences, Engineering, and Medicine). 2020. *Leading Health Indicators 2030: Advancing health, equity, and well-being*. Washington, DC: The National Academies Press. https://doi.org/10.17226/25682.

ODP (Office of Disease Prevention). 2021. *About the ODP*. https://prevention.nih.gov/about-odp/strategic-plan/communicate-efforts-findings (accessed October 22, 2021).

Oeffinger, K. C., E. T. Fontham, R. Etzioni, A. Herzig, J. S. Michaelson, Y. C. Shih, L. C. Walter, T. R. Church, C. R. Flowers, S. J. LaMonte, A. M. Wolf, C. DeSantis, J. Lortet-Tieulent, K. Andrews, D. Manassaram-Baptiste, D. Saslow, R. A. Smith, O. W. Brawley, R. Wender, and American Cancer Society. 2015. Breast cancer screening for women at average risk: 2015 guideline update from the American Cancer Society. *JAMA* 314(15):1599–1614.

Rauh, S., D. Arnold, S. Braga, R. Curca, R. Eckert, A. Frobe, M. Karamouzis, G. Lakatos, and J. L. Molitor. 2018. Challenge of implementing clinical practice guidelines. Getting ESMO's guidelines even closer to the bedside: Introducing the ESMO practising oncologists' checklists and knowledge and practice questions. *ESMO Open* 3(5):e000385.

Truman, B. I., C. K. Smith-Akin, A. R. Hinman, K. M. Gebbie, R. Brownson, L. F. Novick, R. S. Lawrence, M. Pappaioanou, J. Fielding, C. A. Evans, Jr., F. A. Guerra, M. Vogel-Taylor, C. S. Mahan, M. Fullilove, and S. Zaza. 2000. Developing the Guide to Community Preventive Services—overview and rationale: The Task Force on Community Preventive Services. *American Journal of Preventive Medicine* 18(1 Suppl):18–26.

USPSTF (U.S. Preventive Services Task Force). 1989. *Guide to clinical preventive services: An assessment of the effectiveness of 169 interventions: Report of the U.S. Preventive Services Task Force*. Baltimore, MD: Williams & Wilkins. https://wonder.cdc.gov/wonder/prevguid/p0000109/p0000109.asp (accessed November 2, 2021).

USPSTF. 1996. *Guide to clinical preventive services: Report of the U.S. Preventive Services Task Force*. 2nd ed. Washington, DC: U.S. Government Printing Office. https://www.ncbi.nlm.nih.gov/books/NBK15435 (accessed November 2, 2021).

USPSTF. 2002. *Guide to clinical preventive services*. 3rd ed. Rockville, MD: Agency for Healthcare Research and Quality. https://www.ncbi.nlm.nih.gov/books/NBK15199 (accessed November 2, 2021).

USPSTF. 2005. *Guide to clinical preventive services 2005: Recommendations from the U.S. Preventive Services Task Force*. Bethesda, MD: Agency for Healthcare Research and Quality. http://www.lumen.luc.edu/lumen/meded/hmps/pocketgd%5B1%5D.pdf (accessed November 2, 2021).

USPSTF. 2007a. *Guide to clinical preventive services 2007: Recommendations of the U.S. Preventive Services Task Force*. Rockville, MD: Agency for Healthcare Research and Quality. https://www.ncbi.nlm.nih.gov/books/NBK16363 (accessed November 2, 2021).

USPSTF. 2007b. *Motor vehicle occupant restraints: Counseling*. https://www.uspreventiveservicestaskforce.org/uspstf/index.php/recommendation/motor-vehicle-occupant-restraints-counseling (accessed July 19, 2021).

USPSTF. 2008. *Phenylketonuria in newborns: Screening*. https://www.uspreventiveservices-taskforce.org/uspstf/recommendation/phenylketonuria-in-newborns-screening (accessed July 19, 2021).

USPSTF. 2009. *Guide to clinical preventive services 2009: Recommendations of the U.S. Preventive Services Task Force*. Rockville, MD: Agency for Healthcare Research and Quality. https://www.ncbi.nlm.nih.gov/books/NBK37637 (accessed November 2, 2021).

USPSTF. 2010. *Guide to clinical preventive services 2010–2011: Recommendations of the U.S. Preventive Services Task Force*. Rockville, MD: Agency for Healthcare Research and Quality. https://www.ncbi.nlm.nih.gov/books/NBK56707 (accessed November 2, 2021).

USPSTF. 2011. *First annual report to congress on high-priority evidence gaps for clinical preventive services*. https://www.uspreventiveservicestaskforce.org/uspstf/about-uspstf/reports-congress/first-annual-report-congress-high-priority-evidence-gaps-clinical-preventive-services (accessed August 27, 2021).

USPSTF. 2012. *Guide to clinical preventive services 2012: Recommendations of the U.S. Preventive Services Task Force*. Rockville, MD: Agency for Healthcare Research and Quality. https://www.ncbi.nlm.nih.gov/books/NBK115115 (accessed November 2, 2021).

USPSTF. 2014a. *Guide to clinical preventive services 2014: Recommendations of the U.S. Preventive Services Task Force*. Rockville, MD: Agency for Healthcare Research and Quality. https://www.ncbi.nlm.nih.gov/books/NBK235846 (accessed November 2, 2021).

USPSTF. 2014b. *Youth violence: Counseling*. https://www.uspreventiveservicestaskforce.org/uspstf/index.php/recommendation/youth-violence-counseling (accessed July 19, 2021).

USPSTF. 2016. Screening for breast cancer: U.S. Preventive Services Task Force recommendation statement. *Annals of Internal Medicine* 164(4):279–296.

USPSTF. 2017a. *Procedure manual section 6: Methods for arriving at a recommendation*. https://www.uspreventiveservicestaskforce.org/uspstf/about-uspstf/methods-and-processes/procedure-manual/procedure-manual-section-6-methods-arriving-recommendation (accessed July 19, 2021).

USPSTF. 2017b. *Update on methods: Insufficient evidence*. https://www.uspreventiveservicestaskforce.org/uspstf/about-uspstf/methods-and-processes/update-methods-insufficient-evidence (accessed July 19, 2021).

USPSTF. 2018. *Grade definitions*. https://www.uspreventiveservicestaskforce.org/uspstf/about-uspstf/methods-and-processes/grade-definitions (accessed July 19, 2021).

USPSTF. 2019. *Use of decision models in the development of evidence-based clinical preventive services recommendations*. https://www.uspreventiveservicestaskforce.org/uspstf/about-uspstf/methods-and-processes/use-decision-models-development-evidence-based-clinical-preventive-services-recommendations (accessed July 19, 2021).

USPSTF. 2020. *Reports to Congress*. https://www.uspreventiveservicestaskforce.org/uspstf/about-uspstf/reports-congress (accessed July 19, 2021).

USPSTF. 2021a. *About the USPSTF*. https://www.uspreventiveservicestaskforce.org/uspstf/index.php/about-uspstf (accessed July 19, 2021).

USPSTF. 2021b. *Colorectal cancer: Screening*. https://www.uspreventiveservicestaskforce.org/uspstf/recommendation/colorectal-cancer-screening (accessed July 19, 2021).

USPSTF. 2021c. *USPSTF and cost considerations*. https://www.uspreventiveservicestaskforce.org/uspstf/about-uspstf/task-force-resources/uspstf-and-cost-considerations (accessed July 19, 2021).

USPSTF. 2021d. *USPSTF recommendations development process: A graphic overview*. https://www.uspreventiveservicestaskforce.org/uspstf/about-uspstf/methods-and-processes/uspstf-recommendations-development-process-graphic-overview (accessed July 19, 2021).

USPSTF. n.d.-a. *Immunizations for adults*. https://www.uspreventiveservicestaskforce.org/uspstf/index.php/recommendation/immunizations-for-adults (accessed July 19, 2021).

USPSTF. n.d.-b. *Immunizations for children*. https://www.uspreventiveservicestaskforce.org/uspstf/immunizations-children (accessed July 19, 2021).

USPSTF. n.d.-c. *Sickle cell disease (hemoglobinopathies) in newborns: Screening*. https://www.uspreventiveservicestaskforce.org/uspstf/index.php/recommendation/sickle-cell-disease-hemoglobinopathies-in-newborns-screening (accessed July 19, 2021).

USPSTF. n.d.-d. *Understanding how the U.S. Preventive Services Task Force works: USPSTF 101*. https://www.uspreventiveservicestaskforce.org/Home/GetFile/6/91/uspstf101_slides/pdf (accessed July 19, 2021).

Weisz, G., A. Cambrosio, P. Keating, L. Knaapen, T. Schlich, and V. J. Tournay. 2007. The emergence of clinical practice guidelines. *Milbank Quarterly* 85(4):691–727.

Welch, V. A., E. A. Akl, G. Guyatt, K. Pottie, J. Eslava-Schmalbach, M. T. Ansari, H. de Beer, M. Briel, T. Dans, I. Dans, M. Hultcrantz, J. Jull, S. V. Katikireddi, J. Meerpohl, R. Morton, A. Mosdol, J. Petkovic, H. J. Schunemann, R. N. Sharaf, J. A. Singh, R. Stanev, T. Tonia, M. Tristan, S. Vitols, J. Watine, and P. Tugwell. 2017. GRADE equity guidelines 1: Considering health equity in GRADE guideline development: Introduction and rationale. *Journal of Clinical Epidemiology* 90:59–67.

3

Clinical Prevention Research Enterprise

The cornerstone of the U.S. Preventive Services Task Force (USPSTF) recommendations is a review of research related to the preventive screenings and interventions assessed. As described in Chapter 2 and subsequently in Chapter 5, the USPSTF depends on the work of Agency for Healthcare Research and Quality (AHRQ)-funded Evidence-based Practice Centers (EPCs) to identify, assess, and rate the quality of published research findings. This chapter reviews the important role the National Institutes of Health (NIH) serves in funding research relevant to the USPSTF, the contributions of other research funders, and the role of researchers.

NATIONAL INSTITUTES OF HEALTH

Organization and Funding Streams

NIH is an agency of the U.S. Department of Health and Human Services. NIH comprises 27 units, referred to as Institutes and Centers (IC). The Office of the Director sets policy for NIH and plans, manages, and coordinates the work of NIH ICs (NIH, 2021e). The Office of the Director program offices include the Offices of AIDS Research, Behavioral and Social Sciences Research, Disease Prevention, Strategic Coordination, Research on Women's Health, among others. The NIH budget is substantial. Excluding supplemental appropriations for COVID-19 research, the total funding for NIH in fiscal year (FY) 2020 was more than $30 billion

(NIH, 2021e, n.d.-b). NIH supports extramural research, that is, research support to researchers outside the federal government, and intramural research, conducted by NIH employees. In addition, there are collaborative research teams consisting of intramural investigators and extramural researchers from multiple institutions and organizations.

NIH has a multi-layered process for developing its funding priorities (see Box 3-1). The most recent strategic plan identifies three objectives and five crosscutting themes for FY2021–2025 (see Box 3-2). NIH uses a variety of funding mechanisms to achieve its goals. The NIH website lists a total of 245 unique "activity codes" for grants; however, a small handful of these are commonly utilized and well known (NIH, n.d.-a). The R series is for investigator-initiated research projects and the RO1, for example, is the NIH standard independent research project grant mechanism. K awards are research career funding mechanisms. The P award series is for Research Program Projects and Centers. The U series supports cooperative agreements. See Table 3-1 for a description of the most common

BOX 3-1
Setting Research Priorities

Decision makers at NIH seek advice from many sources when setting research priorities:

- The scientific community, including both individual researchers and professional societies;
- Patient organizations and voluntary health associations;
- Institute and Center Advisory Councils;
- Congress and the administration;
- Advisory Committee to the NIH Director (ACD);
- Scientific Management Review Board; and
- NIH staff.

NIH builds its budget by evaluating current opportunities and public health needs while maintaining strong support for investigator-initiated research. The formulation of the NIH budget provides an established framework within which priorities are identified, reviewed, and justified.

A special office was established dedicated to help manage large and complex research portfolios. The Division of Program Coordination, Planning, and Strategic Initiatives identifies important areas of emerging scientific opportunity or rising public health challenges to assist in the acceleration of research investments in these areas.

SOURCE: NIH, 2018b.

BOX 3-2
National Institutes of Health Strategic Plan for Fiscal Years 2021–2025

Key Objectives

- Advancing biomedical and behavioral sciences
- Developing, maintaining, and renewing scientific research capacity
- Exemplifying and promoting the highest level of scientific integrity, public accountability, and social responsibility in the conduct of science

Crosscutting Themes

- Minority health and health disparities
- Women's health
- Public health challenges across the lifespan
- Collaborative science
- Data science

SOURCE: NIH, 2021d.

mechanisms. NIH ICs might vary in which funding mechanisms they use or might have specialized eligibility criteria (NIH, 2019). NIH also issues contracts, which differ from research grants in significant ways, particularly with regard to NIH staff oversight (see Table 3-2).

All awards, whether for grants or contracts, undergo a review process. Most grant applications are subject to peer-review by "study sections." The Center for Scientific Review at NIH reviews 75 percent of all applications to NIH (2021a). Study sections comprise non-NIH experts who serve as recurring or regular members in a particular domain, as well as ad hoc members. Study sections can be either Standing Study Sections or special emphasis panels targeting a specific request for applications. NIH staff experts manage study sections. Study sections evaluate the scientific and technical merit of the proposed research. Individual ICs use these reviews to decide which projects to fund (NIH, 2018b). A minority of applications receive funding. In FY2020, the total number of applications for research project grants and other mechanisms was 75,351. The number of awards was 17,087 for a 22.7 percent "overall success rate" (OER, 2020b). Success rates vary by funding mechanism and by IC. For example, the success rate for RO1s at the National Cancer Institute (NCI) was 12.3 percent but 30.8 percent for the National Heart, Lung, and Blood Institute (NHLBI) PO1 awards.

TABLE 3-1 Frequently Used Funding Mechanisms at the National Institutes of Health

R01	National Institutes of Health (NIH) Research Project Grant Program (R01) • Used to support a discrete, specified, circumscribed research project • NIH's most commonly used grant program • No specific dollar limit unless specified in funding opportunity announcement (FOA) • Advance permission required for $500K or more (direct costs) in any year • Generally awarded for 3–5 years • Utilized by all ICs

R41/R42	Small Business Technology Transfer (STTR)
	• Intended to stimulate scientific and technological innovation through cooperative research/research and development (R/R&D) carried out between small business concerns (SBCs) and research institutions (RIs)
	• Fosters technology transfer between SBCs and RIs
	• Assists the small business and research communities in commercializing innovative technologies
	• Three-phase structure:
	  o I—Feasibility study to establish scientific/technical merit of the proposed R/R&D efforts (generally, 1 year; $150,000)
	  o II—Full R/R&D efforts initiated in phase I (generally 2 years; $1,000,000)
	  o III—Commercialization stage (cannot use STTR funds)
	• Eligibility limited to U.S. small business concerns
	• Project director/principal investigator (PD/PI) may be employed with the SBC *or* the participating nonprofit research institution as long as they has a formal appointment with or commitment to the applicant SBC.
	• Multiple PD/PIs allowed
	• All ICs utilize except Fogarty International Center

TABLE 3-1 Continued

R43/R44	Small Business Innovative Research (SBIR)
	• Intended to stimulate technological innovation in the private sector by supporting R/R&D for for-profit institutions for ideas that have potential for commercialization
	• Assists the small business research community in commercializing innovative technologies
	• Three-phase structure:
	  o I—Feasibility study to establish scientific/technical merit of the proposed R/R&D efforts (generally, 6 months; $150,000)
	  o II—Full research or R&D efforts initiated in phase I (generally 2 years; $1,000,000)
	  o III—Commercialization stage (cannot use SBIR funds)
	• Eligibility limited to U.S. small business concerns
	  o The primary employment of the PD/PI must be with the small business concern
	  o Multiple PD/PIs allowed
	  o All ICs utilize except Fogarty International Center

U01	Research Project Cooperative Agreement • Supports discrete, specified, circumscribed projects to be performed by investigator(s) in an area representing their specific interests and competencies • Used when substantial programmatic involvement is anticipated between the awarding institute and center • One of many types of cooperative agreements • No specific dollar limit unless specified in FOA
P01	Research Program Project Grant • Support for integrated, multi-project research projects involving a number of independent investigators who share knowledge and common resources • Each project contributes or is directly related to the common theme of the total research effort, thus forming a system of research activities and projects directed toward a well-defined research program goal • Specific dollar limit unless specified in FOA

continued

TABLE 3-1 Continued

NIH Common Fund	The Common Fund has been used to support a series of short-term, exceptionally high impact, trans-NIH programs known collectively as the NIH Roadmap for Medical Research. As the Common Fund grows and research opportunities and needs emerge in the scientific community, the portfolio of programs supported by the Common Fund will likely evolve to encompass a diverse set of trans-NIH programs, although the NIH Roadmap is likely to remain a central component. The Other Transaction Authority allows the NIH director to enter into transactions (other than contracts, cooperative agreements, or grants) to carry out research pertaining to the Common Fund. "NIH would use the OTA when it needs greater flexibility to identify and engage nontraditional research partners, or to engage traditional partners in new ways, and negotiate terms and conditions that will concentrate their efforts, spur innovation, and facilitate collaborative problem solving." Typical government procurement and grant laws, regulations, and policies do not apply to OT awards.

SOURCES: Adapted from NIH, 2016b, 2019, n.d.-d.

TABLE 3-2 Comparison of Grants and Contracts

Grant	Contract
Assistance mechanism to support research for the public good	Legally binding agreement to acquire goods or services for the direct use or benefit of the government
Peer review of broad criteria	Award based on peer review of stated evaluation factors, including technical criteria
Limited government oversight and control	More government oversight and control
Reports	Deliverables

SOURCES: Adapted from NIH, 2016a; OER, 2020b.

An NIH summary of funding by grant mechanism from 2011 to 2020 (excluding supplemental COVID-19 appropriations) shows that in FY2019 the vast majority of funding went to research grants (49,092 awards totaling $28.1 billion average award of $573,276), whereas research and development contracts accounted for $1.7 billion (1,188 awards, average award $1,452,924) (OER, 2020a).

National Institutes of Health Solicitation of Research

NIH announces research funding opportunities through the following mechanisms: notice of special interest (NOSI), program announcement (PA), request for application (RFA), request for proposal (RFP), and parent announcements (NIH, 2021b,c, n.d.-c). PAs identify priority areas and usually specify a specific funding mechanism. One subtype, a PAS (a PA with set aside funds), includes funds set aside by an institute or center to fund applications that receive a score beyond the payline (funding cutoff points). Another subtype is known as a PAR, which is a PA whose applications will be reviewed by the funding institute, rather than NIH's Center for Scientific Review. An RFA identifies a narrowly defined area for which one or more institutes has set aside funding for awarding grants (NIH, n.d.-c). RFPs are used to solicit contract proposals. Notices of special interest announce research priorities and direct applicants to PAs.

National Institutes of Health Spending on Prevention Research

In a recent perspective piece the director of the Office of Disease Prevention (ODP) wrote

> Each NIH institute and center defines prevention to reflect its own mission. Even so, a general working definition for research at NIH is this: Prevention research encompasses both primary and secondary prevention. It includes research designed to promote health; to prevent onset of disease, disorders, conditions, or injuries; and to detect, and prevent the progression of, asymptomatic disease. Prevention research targets biology, individual behavior, factors in the social and physical environments, and health services, and informs and evaluates health-related policies and regulations. Prevention research includes studies for the identification and assessment of risk and protective factors; screening and identification of individuals and groups at risk; development and evaluation of interventions to reduce risk; translation, implementation, and dissemination of effective preventive interventions into practice; and development of methods to support prevention research. (Murray, 2017)

Using NIH's Research Portfolio Online Reporting Tool the author noted an upward trend in the number of awards tagged as "prevention" and in the total dollars spent on prevention research between 2010 and 2016 (NIH, n.d.-e). The two ICs with the most money spent on prevention research were the National Institute of Allergy and Infectious Diseases and NCI. Overall, more than 90 percent of 2016 prevention research was funded through the extramural research program, and approximately 14 percent was spent on clinical trials. The author noted challenges to developing a robust prevention research portfolio at NIH, including low success rates, and it is difficult to document the long-term benefits of preventive interventions related to their harms and the number of intervention studies is limited (Murray, 2017). It should be noted that prevention research is a broader category than clinical prevention research and research of direct relevance to the USPSTF is an even more narrow set of research.

Funding of U.S. Preventive Services Task Force–Relevant Clinical Prevention Research

A recent analysis indicates that NIH is the largest single funder of the evidence cited in USPSTF reviews (Villani et al., 2018). The authors reviewed the funding sources for 1,650 articles included in support of 25 recommendations issued by the USPSTF over a 2-year period. Government agencies supported 56 percent of the studies, with nonprofit or university funding second at 32 percent, and industry sponsorship of 17 percent. Funding source was unknown for 21 percent of the studies. The numbers add up to more than 100 percent due to multiple funders for some research publications. NIH contributed funding to 25 percent of the articles, the largest funder identified in that review. A similar review of funding for publications used in support of the work of the Community Preventive Services Task Force, discussed in Chapter 2, showed that NIH was the leading sponsor for effectiveness research and economic reviews (Neilson et al., 2020).

NIH has made significant contributions in sponsoring clinical trials and other research showing the efficacy and effectiveness of clinical preventive interventions, leading to preventive services implemented in practice (Doria-Rose, 2021; Lauer, 2021). For example, the NCI-funded Cancer Intervention and Surveillance Modeling Network, known as CISNET, provides modeling support to the USPSTF upon request. The Population-based Research to Optimize the Screening Process, known as PROSPR, focuses on underserved patient populations, information of great importance to prevention practitioners. The Systolic Blood Pressure Intervention Trial (SPRINT) funded by NHLBI provided important information leading to updated blood pressure guidelines for clinical practice (NIH, n.d.-f).

As discussed in Chapter 2, all USPSTF recommendation statements include a section on research needs and gaps. This committee report was commissioned in part to help make the research needs more actionable. A major focus of the committee has been on those recommendation statements that have an I grade. ODP staff analyzed research that had been instrumental in upgrading an I statement to a letter grade recommendation (Klabunde, 2020; Klabunde et al., 2021). The authors examined 630 research publications cited in the evidence reviews for 14 recommendations that changed from I to a letter grade between 2010 and 2019. The analysis showed that 44 percent of the articles reported results from U.S.-supported studies; NIH provided support for 29 percent of all studies and 62 percent of U.S.-supported studies and was the largest single funder of articles. Thirteen of 27 ICs in NIH provided support. Additional analysis showed that for the NIH-supported studies determined to be "key" for closing nine evidence gaps, three used contract mechanisms, three used only R grants, and three used a combination of funding, including intramural research funding.

The Role of the Office of Disease Prevention

ODP sits in the Division of Program Coordination, Planning, and Strategic Initiatives in the Office of the Director (Murray, 2020). ODP does not have direct grant-making authority and therefore does not issue funding opportunity announcements (FOAs), with the exception of the Tobacco Regulatory Science Program (Klabunde et al., 2021). ODP Strategic Priorities are as follows:

- conduct portfolio analysis and impact assessment,
- identify research gaps,
- improve research methods,
- promote collaborative research,
- advance tobacco regulatory and prevention science, and
- communicate efforts and findings.

It has the following crosscutting themes:

- leading causes and risk factors for premature morbidity and mortality,
- health disparities, and
- dissemination and implementation research.

ODP is the NIH liaison to both the USPSTF and the CPSTF. ODP works with ICs to develop new activities to address gaps identified by both task forces. They use the following methods:

- soliciting IC task force liaisons
- soliciting IC nominations for new task force members
- soliciting IC input for task force topic choices and topic prioritization

- soliciting IC input on proposed task force research plans
- soliciting IC input on task force draft evidence reports and recommendations
- hosting conference calls with AHRQ staff and EPC representatives to discuss I statement research needs and gaps
- convening scientific meetings, workshops, and conferences
- issuing FOAs
- coordinating messaging across NIH for final task force recommendations
- soliciting IC participation in annual I statement survey
- disseminating reports from annual NIH I statement survey

ODP began surveying NIH ICs regarding the activities they have conducted related to I statements since 2015. The I statement survey provides ODP staff information to "identify and advance trans-NIH collaborations to address prevention research gaps." The survey helps AHRQ "plan and prioritize USPSTF preventive services topics" and to demonstrate in its Annual Report to Congress the ways AHRQ and NIH work collaboratively to address critical research gaps in clinical prevention services. In 2015 all 42 current I statements were included in the survey. Beginning in 2018, ODP began collecting information about each I statement every other year on an alternating schedule. Relevant categories for activities include the following:

- active grants
- active contracts
- active Funding Opportunity Announcements
- intramural research projects
- meetings, workshops, and conferences
- publications with new evidence
- collaborations such as interagency agreements and committee or task force memberships

A summary of 2018–2019 current activities documented in the 2020 I statement survey is found in Figure 3-1 and Table 3-3.

For the 26 I statements included in the survey, 22 ICs report activities in 2018 and 2019. It is not obvious from the I statement surveys what proportion these activities represent compared to the totality of activities of each IC, however. In addition to the annual survey, ODP prepares "snapshot" documents for I statements. The I statement for Cognitive Impairment in Older Adults issued in 2020 contains the following research needs (USPSTF, 2020):

- More research is needed on the effect of screening and early detection of cognitive impairment (mild cognitive impairment [MCI] and mild to moderate dementia) on important patient, caregiver, and societal outcomes, including decision making, advance planning, and caregiver outcomes.
- The body of evidence on screening and interventions for cognitive impairment would benefit from more consistent definitions and reporting of outcomes to allow comparisons across trials, especially from trials with longer-term follow-up.
- Studies are needed of the effects of caregiver or patient–caregiver dyad interventions on delay or prevention of institutionalization, and the effects of delay in institutionalization on caregivers.
- Research is needed on treatments that clearly affect the long-term clinical course of cognitive impairment. It is also important that studies on screening and interventions for cognitive impairment report harms and reasons for attrition of trial participants.

I Statements

Results at a Glance 2018–2019

Current Activities	2018	2019
Grants	**832** 22 ICs	**797** 22 ICs
FOAs	**249** 17 ICs	**194** 17 ICs
Contracts	**29** 3 ICs	**29** 3 ICs
Intramural Research Projects	**41** 3 ICs	**41** 4 ICs
Recent Meetings, Workshops, Conferences	**17** 5 ICs	**24** 6 ICs
Publications with New Evidence	**109** 12 ICs	**250** 14 ICs

Survey Summary	
22	Participating ICs
26	I Statements

Other Collaborations	2018	2019
Inter-Agency Agreements	**1** 1 ICs	**1** 1 ICs
Scientific Interest Group Membership	**17** 5 ICs	**18** 5 ICs

FIGURE 3-1 2020 I statement survey summary.
NOTE: FOA = funding opportunity announcement; IC = institute and center.
SOURCE: ODP, 2020a.

TABLE 3-3 National Institutes of Health Activity Related to I Statements

NIH Activity Type	I Statement Topic with the Most NIH-Reported Activity
Grants	• Speech and Language Delay and Disorders in Children Age 5 and Younger: Screening • Cognitive Impairment in Older Adults: Screening
Contracts	• Elevated Blood Lead Levels in Children: Screening • Elevated Blood Lead Levels in Pregnant Women: Screening
FOA	• Lipid Disorders in Children and Adolescents: Screening • Depression in Children and Adolescents: Screening
Intramural Research Project	• Gestational Diabetes Mellitus: Screening • Depression in Children and Adolescents: Screening
Meetings, workshops, conferences	• Depression in Children and Adolescents: Screening • Cognitive Impairment in Older Adults: Screening
Reported publications with new evidence	• Cognitive Impairment in Older Adults: Screening • Autism Spectrum Disorder in Young Children: Screening
Collaborations	• Speech and Language Delay and Disorders in Children Age 5 and Younger: Screening • Lipid Disorders in Children and Adolescents: Screening

SOURCE: Adapted from ODP, 2020a.

The 2020 Snapshot for Cognitive Impairment in Older Adults indicated that 10 ICs reported at least one ongoing activity in 2018 and 2019 (ODP, 2020b). The National Institute on Aging reported the most activities in 2019, including 31 grants, 5 FOAs, 2 meetings/conferences, and 22 publications. Of the total active grants in 2019, 65 were research project grants (R01), 18 were other research grant (R) mechanisms, and 11 were center grants (program project/center [P], career development [K], and cooperative [U] grants). No contracts or intramural projects were identified.

A review of the listed RO1s suggests that research that was considered aligned with the I statement research needs ranges from "Olfactory Receptors for Semiochemical Detection in the Main Olfactory Epithelium" (3 RO1 DC014253-04) to "The UCSF Brain Health Assessment for the Detection of Cognitive Impairment Among Diverse Populations in Primary Care" (UG3NS105557) and "Understanding the Lived Experience of Couples Across the Trajectory of Dementia" (1RO1AG062684-01). Active FOAs range from "Health Disparities and Alzheimer's Disease" (FOA number PAR-15-349) to "Novel Approaches to Diagnosing Alzheimer's Disease and Predicting Progression" (PAR-15-359) and "Central Neural Mechanisms of Age-Related Hearing Loss" (RFA-AG-18-017). Many of the grants, contracts, FOAs, or publications in the Snapshot, while undoubtedly important, would not directly address the Research Needs and Gaps identified by the USPSTF in its 2020 Recommendation Statement. The committee hopes its taxonomy and the recommendations for its use, as described in Chapters 4 and 5, respectively, will offer a structured approach to categorizing research needs.

OTHER CLINICAL PREVENTION RESEARCH FUNDERS

While NIH is the single largest funder of biomedical research in the United States, other funders have an important role to play in clinical prevention research. These include the Centers for Disease Control and Prevention (CDC), the Patient-Centered Outcomes Research Institute (PCORI), the U.S. Department of Veterans Affairs (VA), the U.S. Department of Defense (DOD), voluntary health associations, health systems and payers, and the pharmaceutical and device industries.

Centers for Disease Control and Prevention

CDC has long played a prominent role in prevention of both acute and chronic diseases. CDC supports state and local health departments, conducts research, provides evidence-based advice on important issues, such as vaccination, trains early career clinicians in epidemiologic and outbreak investigations, conducts surveys (i.e., the National Health and Nutrition Examination Survey), on important health topics, runs quarantine stations at ports of entry to the United States, and much more. As discussed in Chapter 2, CDC provides technical and administrative support to the Guide to Community Preventive Services (the Community Guide), a complementary effort to the USPSTF focusing on reviewing evidence for health promotion and disease prevention efforts directed at groups, communities, or other populations (Community Guide, n.d.). A review of the research included in 144 systematic reviews done for the CPSTF shows that while NIH was the leading sponsor of research used in both the effectiveness reviews and the economic reviews, CDC was the second leading sponsor of the research used by the CPSTF (Neilson et al., 2020). CDC was the third highest sponsor of research included in evidence reviews for the USPSTF.

CDC's grant program consists of non-discretionary and discretionary grants, a competitive process. CDC's cooperative agreements are used when it anticipates the need for significant agency involvement. In FY2020 CDC obligated $6.7 billion for non-COVID-19-related activities (CDC, n.d.). CDC funds the Prevention Research Centers (PRCs), teams of academic researchers conducting applied public health prevention research (CDC, 2021). Some of this research is directly linked to topics of interest to the USPSTF but focused on ways to improve the use of preventive services. CDC-funded thematic research networks fund several PRCs to collaborate on a specific issue (CDC, 2020). The Cancer Prevention and Control Research Network includes eight PRCs that conduct research on the "the dissemination and implementation of evidence-based programs proven to increase cancer prevention and control. Members aim to increase the use of these programs among communities and public health partners." (CDC, 2020) Other thematic networks of PRCs with interests complementary to the USPSTF are the Physical Activity Policy Research and Evaluation Network and the Nutrition and Obesity Policy Research and Evaluation Network.

Patient-Centered Outcomes and Research Institute

PCORI has the stated mission to fund "research that offers patients and caregivers the information they need to make important healthcare decisions" (PCORI, 2021a). PCORI's National Priorities are under revision, but the proposed priorities are as follows (PCORI, 2021b):

- Increase Evidence for Existing Interventions and Emerging Innovations in Health
- Enhance Infrastructure to Accelerate Patient-Centered Outcomes Research
- Advance the Science of Dissemination, Implementation, and Health Communication
- Achieve Health Equity
- Accelerate Progress Toward an Integrated Learning Health System

PCORI's FY2019 budget summary shows awards of $147 million for research, $29 million for dissemination and implementation, $25 million for engagement, and $7 million for research infrastructure (PCORI, 2019). PCORI has a program on evidence synthesis, which includes systematic reviews of comparative effectiveness research and other methodologic approaches. PCORI has developed a process by which it prioritizes research funding. The Science Oversight Committee and Advisory Panel uses five criteria (PCORI, 2015):

- **Patient-Centeredness:** Is the comparison relevant to patients, their caregivers, clinicians, or other key stakeholders and are the outcomes relevant to patients?

- **Impact of the Condition on the Health of Individuals and Populations:** Is the condition or disease associated with a significant burden in the U.S. population, in terms of disease prevalence, costs to society, loss of productivity, or individual suffering?
- **Assessment of Current Options:** Does the topic reflect an important evidence gap related to current options that is not being addressed by ongoing research?
- **Likelihood of Implementation in Practice:** Would new information generated by research be likely to have an impact in practice? (E.g., do one or more major stakeholder groups endorse the question?)
- **Durability of Information:** Would new information on this topic remain current for several years, or would it be rendered obsolete quickly by new technologies or subsequent studies?

U.S. Department of Veterans Affairs

The VA's nationwide electronic health records lends itself to adhering to preventive interventions recommended by the USPSTF (Atkins, 2021). These 9 million records may be useful for addressing certain evidence gaps. In addition, the VA, where needed, will invest in large, definitive, national trials. For example, the CONFIRM study includes 50,000 veterans randomized to colonoscopy or to annual fecal immunochemical testing (FIT) who will be followed for 10 years to assess cancer incidence and mortality (VA, 2017). The PIVOT trial, a collaboration among the VA, NCI, and AHRQ, compared surgery versus watchful waiting for low-risk prostate cancer (Wilt, 2012). When considering priority gaps as a funder, the VA asks the following:

- Is it an important problem for their population?
- Is this an intervention they can deliver at scale if effective?
- Is the VA a logical place for a trial?
- Could VA population-based electronic health records data answer the question without a prospective randomized controlled trial? (Atkins, 2021).

U.S. Department of Defense

DOD was the second-largest federal sponsor of medical and health research and development in 2017, spending more than $2 billion (CRS, 2019; Research!America, 2018). Spending on health research at DOD goes through two distinct appropriations, the standard appropriations process and the Congressionally Directed Medical Research Program

(CDMRP) (Mendez, 2020). This funding is used only for medical research on topics identified by Congress. In FY2020 its budget was $1.4 billion and has accounted in recent years for at least half of the Defense Health Program's Research, Development, Test, and Evaluation budget. Historically the largest research programs addressed breast cancer, prostate cancer, psychological health and traumatic brain injury, and two general programs for peer-reviewed medical research and peer-reviewed cancer research. In addition to the CDMRP priorities DOD health research includes the following focus areas: biomedical informatics and health information systems and technology, clinical and rehabilitative medicine, combat casualty care, medical chemical and biological defense, medical radiological defense, military infectious diseases, and military operational medicine (DOD, 2019). The single largest component of the Defense Health Program is TRICARE, the health care insurance program for more than 9 million service members, retirees, and beneficiaries (MHS, n.d.). Non-DOD researchers are subject to requirements for using the Military Health System data beyond the requirements for DOD investigators (OASDHA, 2012).

Health Systems

While the VA is among the largest health systems that sponsors research, many other health systems fund or host research. For example, the Health Care Systems Research Network includes 19 health systems with embedded research groups that are generally funded by a combination of internal and external sponsors (HCSRN, 2021; Rahm et al., 2019). Some systems, including Kaiser Permanente, HealthPartners, Intermountain Healthcare, and the Hospital Corporation of America, have invested substantial amounts of internal funding in applied research, which involves evaluating clinical or organizational practices that health systems can implement or encourage (Lieu and Platt, 2017).

Health systems also serve as environments for studies sponsored by NIH and other external funders that enable improved clinical decision making and identify care processes that improve safety, efficacy and effectiveness. For example, NIH has sponsored studies of how real-life factors, such as physician performance and patient adherence, influence the effectiveness of colonoscopy and fecal immunochemical testing in large-scale programs for colorectal cancer screening. NIH's Health Care Systems Research Collaboratory is another large-scale effort that engages organizations including clinics and hospitals in pragmatic clinical trials, aiming to generate real-world evidence on benefits and risks of treatment options (NIH, 2018a). Whether funded internally or externally, research on dissemination and implementation conducted in health systems can be directly applied to guide the development of real-world programs in clinical prevention.

Voluntary Health Associations

A recent analysis indicates that voluntary health organizations contribute less than 1 percent of all health research funds; however, those funds are far from trivial (Research!America, 2018). For example, in 2018 the American Cancer Society reported expenses of almost $148 million toward cancer research, second only to NIH (ACA, 2019; McKenzie et al., 2018). In 2019 the American Diabetes Association reported spending almost $37 million for research (ADA, 2019). A particularly important type of research funded by these types of organizations is for implementation of research findings, although they do provide support for clinical trials. Another major contribution of voluntary health agencies is their advocacy for funding for research (McKenzie et al., 2018).

Private Industry

Private industry funds a significant amount of biomedical research in the United States. The analysis of who funds the research cited in USPSTF systematic reviews indicated that 17 percent of articles were funded in full or in part by industry (Villani et al., 2018). Of the recommendation topics reviewed, screening for chlamydia and gonorrhea had the highest proportion of papers funded by industry (75 percent). Several of the preventive interventions are either directly of relevance to the pharmaceutical industry (preventive medications) or indirectly (screening for a condition whose treatment involves a pharmaceutical or device); thus industry is an obvious partner in evidence generation for USPSTF use.

International Sources of Funding

As described earlier, research into the source of funding for research articles included in the systematic reviews used by the USPSTF indicates that NIH is the largest government contributor (420 articles). However, the USPSTF does not restrict itself to research funded by or conducted in the United States. The United Kingdom provided funding for 84 articles, the National Health and Medical Research Council of Australia supported research in 37 articles, and the Netherlands Organisation for Health Research and Development supported research in 35 articles (Villani et al., 2018).

RESEARCHERS

Generating a body of evidence aimed toward addressing an evidence gap often requires research that spans multiple disciplines and areas of expertise. For example, clinical experts are needed specific to adult or pediatric patients, and within these broad categories, to address specific subspecialties (e.g., cardiology, cancer, mental health). In addition, expertise may be needed in health services research, biostatistics, modeling, clinical trial design, and economics. Such a team may require multiple institutions to include the researchers best equipped to design and conduct a study that generates the needed evidence.

The inclusion of multiple institutions may also be needed to address evidence gaps in specific populations, such as racial/ethnic minorities and/or persons at high risk for the condition. The inclusion of these groups reduces health inequities and improves the generalizability of the generated evidence. Moreover, studies conducted at multiple institutions in different settings provide important context about how clinical prevention services manifest in academic medical centers, in community settings (including safety net settings), and in different health care delivery organizations, such as integrated health care systems. Researchers need to have the flexibility to convene such teams and may even be encouraged to do so. NIH has a track record of incentivizing teams such as CISNET and the former Cancer Research Network for the purpose of generating evidence within or across specific research settings. An advantage of these collaborative research arrangements is the investment in infrastructure and expertise that may facilitate future research in a more expedient, nimble manner.

Researchers can play an important role in drafting and reviewing funding announcements through their participation on NIH advisory panels (e.g., NCI convenes a panel of researchers to identify provocative questions and also has a Board of Scientific Advisors). A collaborative relationship between the research community and funders can help to ensure that submitted applications meet the intent of the research call. This exchange will also inform funders about the time required to respond to such calls for applications so that multi-institutional and multidisciplinary groups can contractually come together and meet regulatory requirements, such as an institutional review board review.

REFERENCES

ACA (American Cancer Society). 2019. *2018 Annual Report.* https://www.cancer.org/content/dam/cancer-org/online-documents/en/pdf/reports/2018-annual-report.pdf (accessed November 2, 2021).

ADA (American Diabetes Association). 2019. *2019 Annual Report.* Arlington, VA: American Diabetes Association. https://www.diabetes.org/sites/default/files/2021-01/ADA-2019-AnnualReport.pdf (accessed November 2, 2021).

Atkins, D. 2021. *Funder perspectives on addressing evidence gaps.* Presented on March 16, 2021, at Meeting 4 of the Committee on Addressing Evidence Gaps in Clinical Prevention. https://www.nationalacademies.org/event/03-16-2021/addressing-evidence-gaps-in-clinical-prevention-committee-meeting-session-2 (accessed November 2, 2021).

CDC (Centers for Disease Control and Prevention). 2020. *Thematic research networks.* https://www.cdc.gov/prc/thematic-networks.htm (accessed August 30, 2021).

CDC. 2021. *Prevention research centers.* https://www.cdc.gov/prc/index.htm (accessed August 30, 2021).

CDC. n.d. *Office of the Financial Resources (OFR) FY-2020 assistance snapshot at CDC.* https://www.cdc.gov/funding/documents/fy2020/fy-2020-ofr-assistance-snapshot-508.pdf (accessed August 30, 2021).

Community Guide. n.d. *About the Community Guide.* https://www.thecommunityguide.org/about/about-community-guide (accessed August 30, 2021).

CRS (Congressional Research Service). 2019. *FY-2020 budget request for the Military Health System.* https://sgp.fas.org/crs/natsec/IF11206.pdf (accessed August 30, 2021).

DOD (U.S. Department of Defense). 2019. *Department of Defense strategic medical research plan response to Section 736 of the John S. McCain National Defense Authorization Act for fiscal year 2019 (Public Law 115-232).* https://health.mil/Reference-Center/Congressional-Testimonies/2019/04/08/Strategic-Medical-Research-Plan (accessed August 31, 2021).

Doria-Rose, V. P. 2021. *Pathways to understanding evidence gaps: Funders' perspective.* Presented on March 4, 2021, at Meeting 4 of the Committee on Addressing Evidence Gaps in Clinical Prevention. https://www.nationalacademies.org/event/03-04-2021/addressing-evidence-gaps-in-clinical-prevention-committee-meeting-4-session-1 (accessed October 26, 2021).

HCSRN (Health Care Systems Research Network). 2021. *Health care systems research network: Membership.* https://www.hcsrn.org/en/About/Membership (accessed August 30, 2021).

Klabunde, C. N. 2020. *Engaging NIH and extramural investigators in addressing evidence gaps in clinical prevention.* Presented on December 15, 2020, at Meeting 1 of the Committee on Addressing Evidence Gaps in Clinical Prevention.https://www.nationalacademies.org/event/12-15-2020/addressing-evidence-gaps-in-clinical-prevention-committee-meeting-1-session-2 (accessed November 2, 2021).

Klabunde, C. N., E. M. Ellis, J. Villani, E. Neilson, K. Schwartz, E. A. Vogt, and Q. Ngo-Metzger. 2021. Characteristics of scientific evidence informing changed U.S. Preventive Services Task Force insufficient evidence statements. *American Journal of Preventive Medicine.* https://www.sciencedirect.com/science/article/abs/pii/S0749379721004578 (accessed November 29, 2021).

Lauer, M. 2021. *Perspectives on addressing evidence gaps: NIH.* Presented on March 16, 2021, at Meeting 4 of the Committee on Addressing Evidence Gaps in Clinical Prevention. https://www.nationalacademies.org/event/03-16-2021/addressing-evidence-gaps-in-clinical-prevention-committee-meeting-session-2 (accessed October 26, 2021).

Lieu, T. A., and R. Platt. 2017. Applied research and development in health care—Time for a frameshift. *New England Journal of Medicine* 376(8):710–713. https://www.nejm.org/doi/full/10.1056/nejmp1611611 (accessed November 2, 2021).

McKenzie, J. F., R. R. Pinger, and D. Seabert. 2018. Organizations that help shape community and public health. In *An introduction to community & public health.* 9th ed. Burlington, MA: Jones & Bartlett Learning.

Mendez, B. H. P. 2020. *Congressionally directed medical research programs: Background and issues for Congress.* Washington, DC: Congressional Research Service. https://www.everycrsreport.com/files/2020-11-10_R46599_76afd8a7d9eef054e19c53392f97485ff7b3037e.pdf (accessed November 2, 2021).

MHS (Military Health System). n.d. *Patients by beneficiary category.* https://www.health.mil/I-Am-A/Media/Media-Center/Patient-Population-Statistics/Patients-by-Beneficiary-Category (accessed August 30).

Murray, D. M. 2017. Prevention research at the National Institutes of Health. *Public Health Reports* 132(5):535–538.

Murray, D. 2020. *Closing evidence gaps in clinical prevention: A perspective from the NIH.* Presented on December 15, 2020, at Meeting 1 of the Committee on Addressing Evidence Gaps in Clinical Prevention. https://www.nationalacademies.org/event/12-15-2020/addressing-evidence-gaps-in-clinical-prevention-committee-meeting-1-session-2 (accessed November 2, 2021).

Neilson, E., J. Villani, S. L. Mercer, D. L. Tilley, I. Vincent, A. Alston, and C. N. Klabunde. 2020. Sources of support for studies that inform recommendations of the Community Preventive Services Task Force. *Public Health Reports* 135(6):813–822.

NIH (National Institutes of Health). 2016a. *Contracts.* https://grants.nih.gov/funding/contracts.htm (accessed November 2, 2021).

NIH. 2016b. Frequently asked questions for other transaction awards. *All of Us Research Program.* https://www.nih.gov/allofus-research-program/frequently-asked-questions-other-transaction-awards (accessed November 2, 2021).

NIH. 2018a. *HCS research collaboratory—Demonstration projects for pragmatic clinical trials (ug3/uh3) rfa-rm-16-019.* https://commonfund.nih.gov/hcscollaboratory/fundedresearch (accessed August 30, 2021).

NIH. 2018b. *NIH research planning.* https://www.nih.gov/about-nih/nih-research-planning (accessed August 11, 2021).

NIH. 2019. *Types of grant programs.* https://grants.nih.gov/grants/funding/funding_program.htm (accessed August 11, 2021).

NIH. 2021a. *About CSR.* https://public.csr.nih.gov/AboutCSR (accessed August 11, 2021).

NIH. 2021b. *Funding types: Know the differences.* https://www.ninds.nih.gov/Funding/About-Funding/Funding-Types-Know-Differences (accessed August 30, 2021).

NIH. 2021c. *NIH guide for grants and contracts.* https://grants.nih.gov/funding/searchguide/index.html (accessed August 30, 2021).

NIH. 2021d. *NIH-wide strategic plan.* https://www.nih.gov/about-nih/nih-wide-strategic-plan (accessed November 2, 2021).

NIH. 2021e. *Who we are.* https://www.nih.gov/about-nih/who-we-are/organization (accessed August 10, 2021).

NIH. n.d.-a. *Activity codes search results.* https://grants.nih.gov/grants/funding/ac_search_results.htm (accessed August 10, 2021).

NIH. n.d.-b. *Budget and spending.* https://report.nih.gov/funding/nih-budget-and-spending-data-past-fiscal-years/budget-and-spending (accessed August 10, 2021).

NIH. n.d.-c. *Description of the NIH guide for grants and contracts.* https://grants.nih.gov/grants/guide/description.htm (accessed August 30, 2021).

NIH. n.d.-d. *NIH Common Fund and other transaction authority.* https://dpcpsi.nih.gov/sites/default/files/OTA_slide_508.pdf (accessed November 2, 2021).

NIH. n.d.-e. *RePORTER.* https://report.nih.gov (accessed August 11, 2021).

NIH. n.d.-f. *Systolic blood pressure intervention trial (SPRINT) study.* https://www.nhlbi.nih.gov/science/systolic-blood-pressure-intervention-trial-sprint-study (accessed October 26, 2021).

OASDHA (Office of the Assistant Secretary of Defense for Health Affairs). 2012. *Guide for DOD researchers on MHS data.* Washington, DC: U.S. Department of Defense. https://health.mil/Reference-Center/Publications/2012/10/10/Guide-for-DoD-Researchers-on-Using-MHS-Data (accessed November 2, 2021).

ODP (Office of Disease Prevention). 2020a. *NIH activities related to "insufficient evidence" statements of the US Preventive Services Task Force: Results from the 2020 annual survey of institutes, centers, and offices. Attachment from personal correspondence with Carrie Klabunde, AHRQ staff member, January 7, 2021.* Available by request from the project Public Access File at https://www8.nationalacademies.org/pa/ManageRequest.aspx?key=51932 (accessed November 3, 2021).

ODP. 2020b. *Snapshot of I statement survey results: Cognitive impairment in older adults: Screening. Attachment from personal correspondence with Carrie Klabunde, AHRQ staff member, January 8, 2021.* Available by request from the project Public Access File at https://www8.nationalacademies.org/pa/ManageRequest.aspx?key=51932 (accessed November 3, 2021).

OER (Office of Extramural Research). 2020a. *NIH research grants and other mechanisms including research and development contracts.* https://report.nih.gov/funding/nih-budget-and-spending-data-past-fiscal-years/budget-and-spending (accessed November 2, 2021).

OER. 2020b. *Research project grants (RPGs) and other mechanisms. Table #205C.* https://report.nih.gov/funding/nih-budget-and-spending-data-past-fiscal-years/success-rates (accessed November 2, 2021).

PCORI (Patient-Centered Outcomes Research Institute). 2015. *Generation and prioritization of topics for funding announcements.* https://www.pcori.org/research-results/how-we-select-research-topics/generation-and-prioritization-topics-funding-4 (accessed August 30, 2021).

PCORI. 2019. *PCORI 2019 report.* Washington, DC: Patient-Centered Outcomes Research Insitute. https://www.pcori.org/2019-annual-report (accessed November 2, 2021).

PCORI. 2021a. *Our programs.* https://www.pcori.org/about-us/our-programs (accessed August 11, 2021).

PCORI. 2021b. *PCORI's proposed national priorities for health: An ambitious vision for the years ahead.* https://www.pcori.org/blog/proposed-national-priorities-for-health-an-ambitious-vision-for-the-years-ahead (accessed August 30, 2021).

Rahm, A. K., I. Ladd, A. N. Burnett-Hartman, M. M. Epstein, J. T. Lowery, C. Y. Lu, P. A. Pawloski, R. N. Sharaf, S. Y. Liang, and J. E. Hunter. 2019. The Healthcare Systems Research Network (HCSRN) as an environment for dissemination and implementation research: A case study of developing a multi-site research study in precision medicine. *eGEMs* 7(1):16.

Research!America. 2018. *U.S. investments in medical and health research and development 2013–2017.* https://www.researchamerica.org/sites/default/files/Policy_Advocacy/2013-2017InvestmentReportFall2018.pdf (accessed August 30, 2021).

USPSTF (U.S. Preventive Services Task Force). 2020. *Cognitive impairment in older adults: Screening.* https://www.uspreventiveservicestaskforce.org/uspstf/recommendation/cognitive-impairment-in-older-adults-screening (accessed August 17, 2021).

VA (U.S. Department of Veterans Affairs). 2017. *Largest-ever VA clinical trial enrolls 50,000th* veteran. https://www.research.va.gov/currents/1117-Largest-ever-VA-clinical-trial.cfm (accessed November 2, 2021).

Villani, J., Q. Ngo-Metzger, I. S. Vincent, and C. N. Klabunde. 2018. Sources of funding for research in evidence reviews that inform recommendations of the US Preventive Services Task Force. *JAMA* 319(20):2132–2133.

Wilt, T. J. 2012. The prostate cancer intervention versus observation trial: VA/NCI/AHRQ cooperative studies program #407 (PIVOT): Design and baseline results of a randomized controlled trial comparing radical prostatectomy with watchful waiting for men with clinically localized prostate cancer. *Journal of the National Cancer Institute Monographs* 2012(45):184–190.

4

Taxonomy and Workflow

The heart of the committee's assignment, as described in the Statement of Task (see Box 1-1), was to "develop a taxonomy of [clinical prevention] evidence gaps." This chapter describes the taxonomy that the committee developed and offers examples of how that taxonomy can be applied to describe evidence gaps in clinical prevention research. In particular, it describes the taxonomy as it relates to recommendations and I statements issued by the U.S. Preventive Services Task Force (USPSTF) in its efforts to characterize what is known about the effectiveness of various preventive services in particular populations.

The need for a taxonomy of research gaps in preventive medicine is best understood in terms of the current situation facing the USPSTF. As described in Chapter 2, the 16-member USPSTF reviews the scientific evidence related to various clinical preventive services and then makes evidence-based conclusions about the benefits of these services. The USPSTF offers recommendations for screenings, preventive medications, and behavioral counseling accompanied by a letter grade indicating the magnitude and degree of certainty of the net benefit of the service based on the evidence. In the case of an A recommendation, for instance, the USPSTF recommends the preventive service and has concluded that "there is high certainty that the net benefit is substantial" (USPSTF, 2018c). A B recommendation would also indicate that the USPSTF recommends the service, but that there is either "high certainty that the net benefit is moderate or there is moderate certainty that the net benefit is moderate to substantial." A C recommendation indicates that the USPSTF recommends that clinicians selectively offer a service based on their "professional judgment and patient preferences" as "there is at least moderate certainty the net benefit is small." A D recommendation indicates that the USPSTF discourages a particular preventive service, as there is "moderate to high certainty that the service has no net benefit or that the harms outweigh the benefits."

Some services may also receive an I statement, which is a non-recommendation, and indicates that the USPSTF could not find sufficient evidence to make a recommendation either for or against the service. I statements indicate that the USPSTF has concluded that "the current evidence [regarding the service] is insufficient to assess the balance of benefits and harms of the service. Evidence is lacking, of poor quality, or conflicting, and the balance of benefits and harms cannot be determined" (USPSTF, 2018c).

As of September 14, 2021, there are 86 published topics that have at least one letter grade recommendation or I statement. Out of 131 individual letter grade recommendations or I statements issued across the 86 topics, 53 are I statements (encompassing 46 topics) (see Appendix A). Some cover an entire preventive topic, such as screening the general population for celiac disease, where the USPSTF has concluded that there is not enough evidence to make a recommendation one way or the other (USPSTF, 2017). In other cases, the I statement relates to a particular population, as with the recommendation for screening for chlamydia and gonorrhea: the USPSTF recommends screening women with a B grade but issued an I statement regarding screening men (USPSTF, 2021b).

The U.S. Department of Health and Human Services developed the USPSTF to issue clinical practice guidelines based on the existing medical literature, with little to no focus on assessing evidence gaps. In the intervening decades, Agency for Healthcare Research and Quality (AHRQ) staff and the USPSTF have increasingly prioritized identification of evidence gaps in each recommendation statement with the goal of catalyzing clinical prevention research on those topics. Additionally, the Office of Disease Prevention (ODP) liaises with National Institutes of Health (NIH) institutes and centers to make evidence gaps identified by the USPSTF known across NIH. However, the potential synergy between the USPSTF recommendations and the clinical prevention research community remains unrealized: recommendation updates are published about every 5 years, but a recent paper by Klabunde et al. (2021) observes that, on average, 8.4 years elapse between an I statement and a definitive recommendation being published. This is the state of affairs that the USPSTF, AHRQ, and NIH would like to change, and it is the issue that this report is intended to address.

Closing the evidence gaps in I statements would allow the USPSTF to give guidance to clinicians in areas where uncertainty now reigns and thus improve health outcomes for many different groups of people. Another issue is that any topic with a letter grade recommendation may also have evidence gaps. It would be valuable as well to identify those areas in order to strengthen the evidence base for clinical preventive services more broadly.

Because the USPSTF neither conducts original research nor funds research conducted by others, it cannot directly address these evidence gaps. However, it can recast the evidence gaps sections of its recommendation statements to improve the likelihood that clinical prevention researchers will fill in the gaps. As NIH wrote in the request for proposal to the National Academies of Sciences, Engineering, and Medicine that resulted in this study, "More rigorous or systematic categorization of evidence gaps through application of a taxonomy may help stakeholders better understand and use the evidence gaps, assess their relative importance, identify innovative methods to help fill the evidence gaps, and accelerate research that addresses evidence gaps." This is the purpose of the taxonomy described in this chapter.

As noted in that request for proposal, the taxonomy is intended to assist a number of different groups of stakeholders, including the following:

- Organizations that develop preventive services recommendations, such as the USPSTF, to more clearly communicate evidence gaps.
- Funding agencies, including NIH, to understand, assess the relative importance of, and use evidence gaps from preventive services recommendations in order to ultimately support research to fill the gaps.
- Members of the research community to focus their research on high-priority areas that have evidence gaps.
- All stakeholders to bridge the translation of evidence gaps into funding opportunities and other initiatives that ultimately use innovative methods to close evidence gaps related to clinical preventive services.

Ultimately, the main contribution of the taxonomy is to provide a structured approach to describing evidence gaps related to preventive services so that recommendations and I statements can be thorough and consistent in how they list and describe those gaps. The taxonomy serves as a road map, providing a systematic, step-by-step approach to the characterization of evidence gaps to supplement or replace the more subjective and less systematic descriptions that are currently found in USPSTF recommendations and I statements. Standardizing the process of describing evidence gaps should help increase the consistency and thoroughness of the USPSTF's efforts and make the recommendation statements more clear and consistent for researchers who are interested in helping to fill in evidence gaps.

To provide a clear and thorough explanation of the taxonomy the committee developed for use by the USPSTF, this chapter begins with a description of the approach that the committee took in creating the taxonomy, including an overview of taxonomies in general and a discussion of why the committee chose the particular type of taxonomy it did. Next is a section on the broader framework that the committee developed in which the taxonomy is applied. As will be explained in more detail in that section, the committee sees the taxonomy as something that is applied not in isolation but as part of a larger effort to characterize, understand, and prioritize evidence gaps and develop a research agenda for addressing those gaps. Thus the development of a taxonomy is just one step in this larger task.

With this framework having been described, the next section goes into detail about using the taxonomy to characterize evidence gaps, while the following section discusses how those evidence gaps might be prioritized and a research agenda created that will fill in those gaps according to the prioritization. A final section offers illustrations of how the taxonomy might be applied to specific I statements.

COMMITTEE'S APPROACH

The committee developed and honed its taxonomy and accompanying workflow over many months of research and discussion. One of the first steps was to carry out a literature search on taxonomies to develop a clear idea of what a taxonomy is and how it is used. The committee also worked to understand exactly what was being asked of them in the statement of task; this part of the process involved having conversations with the study's sponsors as well as soliciting input from outside experts. In addition, the committee convened four public meetings to discuss the various issues and problems related to the USPSTF recommendation statements as well as to hear suggestions for the best ways to address these issues.

Understanding Taxonomies

Taxonomies come in various forms, but they all share certain characteristics. The general purpose of any taxonomy, for instance, is to bring order to a collection of information by organizing and systematizing it with a fixed vocabulary and clearly defined structure. A well-designed taxonomy makes it easier to see the big picture and to think about and work with the mass of information that it has imposed order on. Thus the committee investigated a multitude of types of taxonomies to decide which would be most appropriate for the task of organizing and characterizing evidence gaps concerning clinical preventive services.

A taxonomy refers to "any controlled vocabulary of terms for a subject area domain or a specific purpose. The terms may or may not be arranged in a hierarchy, and they may or may not have even more complex relationships between each other" (Hedden, 2016, p. xxiv). The most well-known modern type of taxonomy is the Linnaean taxonomy used to classify living organisms. It has a tree-like branching structure with kingdoms broken into phyla, which are divided into classes, which are subdivided into orders, which are even further subdivided into families, genera, and species. In such hierarchical taxonomies, each item—other than those at the very top or bottom levels—has a broader "parent" category to which it belongs and contains one or more "child" classifications. These taxonomies are common and are used to organize not only living organisms but also such things as books in a library or pages in a website.

However, not all collections of information can be organized in such a hierarchical taxonomy. Information specialists have devised a variety of other approaches to organizing information, which can be characterized in three broad types of knowledge organization systems:

1. Term lists (authority files, glossaries, dictionaries);
2. Classifications and categories (subject headings, hierarchical taxonomies, categorization schemes); and
3. Relationship lists (thesauri, semantic networks, and ontologies) (Hedden, 2016, p. 2).

Traditionally, many of these knowledge organization systems were not referred to as "taxonomies"—that term was strictly for the hierarchical taxonomy and often specifically for the organization of living organisms—but since the 1990s "taxonomy" has come to be used by information specialists to describe knowledge organization systems in general. Additionally, taxonomy documents are living documents, which should be updated regularly to incorporate new concepts and elements as needed.

In learning about taxonomies and thinking about which would be most appropriate to apply to evidence gaps in preventive services, the committee decided the traditional hierarchical taxonomy was not an appropriate system to identify and categorize evidence gaps in clinical prevention, which required the allowance of multiple nested terms. Instead, the committee selected a faceted taxonomy, a type of polyhierarchical taxonomy. Because of the structure of this faceted taxonomy, evidence gaps may be localized informally while the USPSTF develops a recommendation statement, and specified later with the nested terms within the facets. The important feature of the taxonomy is that it provides a systematic method and language for identifying and describing the various gaps in evidence relating to clinical preventive services.

Adapting the U.S. Preventive Services Task Force Analytic Framework

In its search for a suitable taxonomy, the committee examined various potential choices. It looked, for instance, at the PICOTS (population, intervention, comparator, outcome, timing, setting) framework but decided that while this is an effective approach to characterizing an individual research study, it was not a particularly suitable framework for characterizing evidence gaps. As it worked through the different possibilities, the committee decided that the taxonomy should be straightforward; researchers with no particular expertise in information sciences should be able to understand, apply, and utilize it to identify evidence gaps.

Ultimately, after considering various approaches, the committee decided that the analytic framework used by the USPSTF to assess the evidence base and issue a recommendation would also serve to guide its analysis of evidence gaps. To supplement the evidence gap categories related to the analytic framework, the committee added two other facets of the taxonomy: "foundational issues" and "dissemination and implementation" (D&I). Partly in recognition of the USPSTF's commitment to promoting health equity (Davidson et al., 2020, 2021; Doubeni et al., 2021), the committee has made an effort to highlight how the taxonomy and workflow can contribute to the promotion of health equity.

A USPSTF analysis using the analytic framework begins with the specification of a population at risk of a preventable disease or condition, and examines the evidence for links between particular actions (screening, prevention efforts, treatment) and particular outcomes (early detection, decreased morbidity or mortality, adverse effects, etc.). Each line in the figure between an action and an outcome is associated with a question of interest, for example,

- Does screening lead to an early detection of the target condition?
- Does screening lead to adverse effects?
- Do early detection and treatment lead to reduced morbidity or mortality?
- Do early detection and treatment lead to an intermediate outcome that may in turn be related to a decrease in morbidity or mortality?
- Do early detection and treatment lead to adverse effects?

It is important to note that the evidence base addressing these key questions typically provides for two "generic" analytic frameworks for screening and behavioral interventions (see Figures 4-1 and 4-2), which outline the overall approach to developing key questions about linkages. See Figures 4-3 and 4-4 for more complex frameworks developed by the USPSTF to address specific topics (e.g., preventing dental caries among children younger than age 5 and recommending preexposure prophylaxis [PrEP]). When the USPSTF examines the evidence concerning the effectiveness of a preventive service, it uses these questions to guide its analysis and to frame the reporting of its results.

The committee decided that these main components of the analytic framework—the risk assessment, early detection, intermediate outcomes, effectiveness, harms—could serve as ideal building blocks of the taxon-

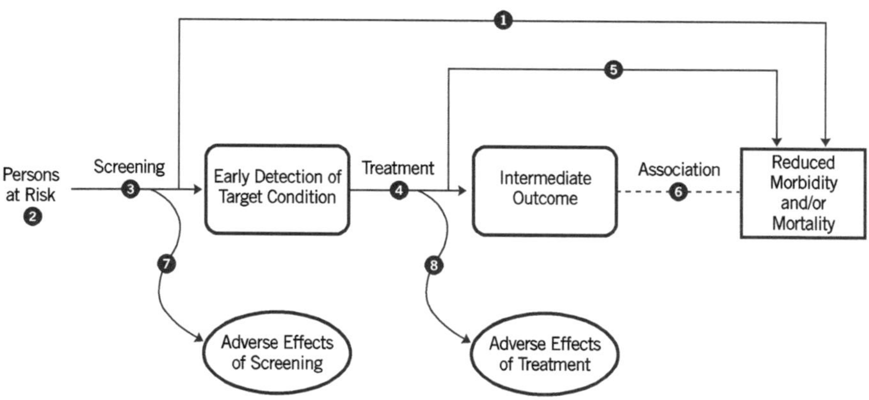

FIGURE 4-1 Generic analytic framework for screenings.
SOURCE: USPSTF, 2021c.

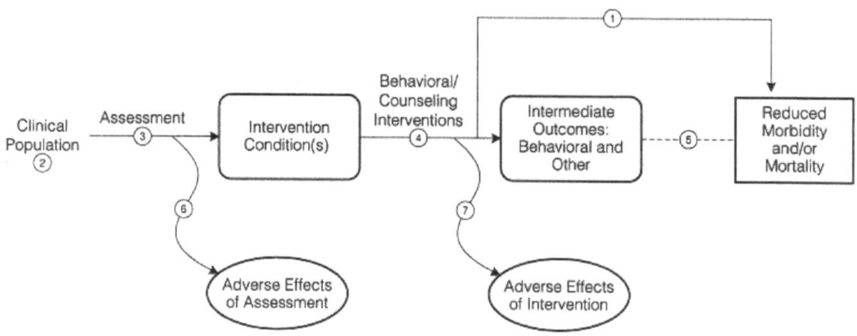

FIGURE 4-2 Generic analytic framework for behavioral interventions.
SOURCE: Harris et al., 2001.

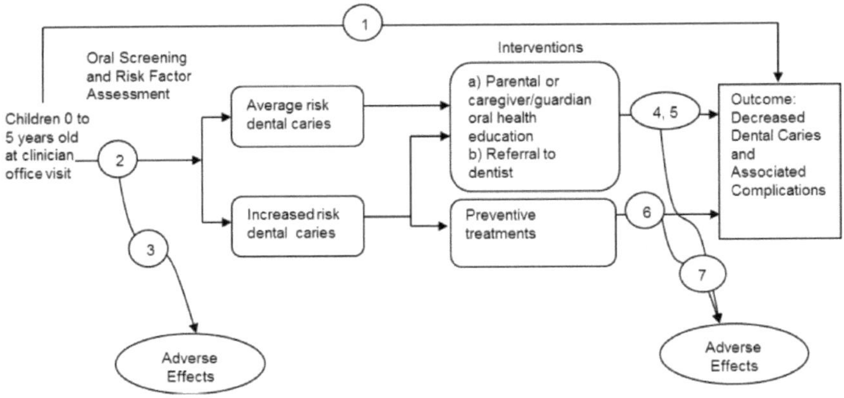

FIGURE 4-3 Analytic framework for screenings and interventions to prevent dental caries in children younger than age 5.
SOURCE: Chou et al., 2014.

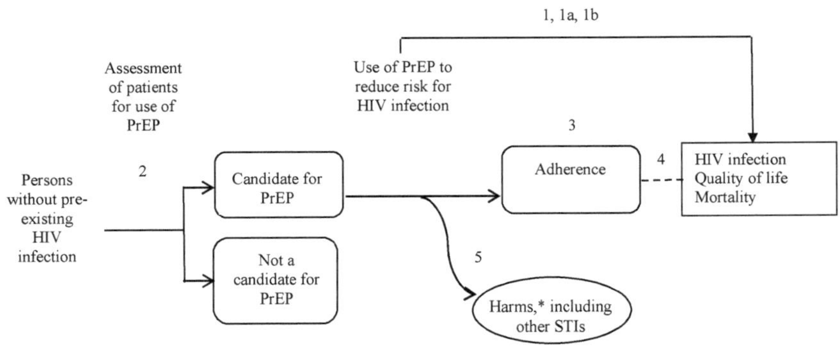

FIGURE 4-4 Analytic framework for preventing HIV infection with PrEP.
NOTE: PrEP = preexposure prophylaxis; STI = sexually transmitted infection.
SOURCE: Chou et al., 2019.

omy, allowing the USPSTF to identify those evidence gaps that are most relevant to their evaluations. However, the committee determined that a taxonomy consisting only of elements from the analytic framework would be incomplete; thus they added other components to fill it out.

Evidence gap categories related to the foundational issues facet are often already recognized by the USPSTF. For example, the USPSTF has issued an I statement for screening for glaucoma. The USPSTF (2013) notes, "The natural history of glaucoma, particularly the role of IOP [intraocular pressure] and its relationship to optic nerve damage, visual field defects, visual impairment, and blindness, is poorly understood." While other evidence gaps address questions directly related to risk assessment, benefits, harms, intermediate outcomes, and health outcomes, some address more foundational elements of a disease (e.g., its natural history). Many foundational evidence gaps are coupled with analytic framework gaps in the USPSTF recommendations and I statements, and not all foundational evidence gaps will need to be addressed before analytic gaps are addressed. However, foundational gaps are distinct from the analytic framework gaps because they do not directly address linkages between actions and outcomes.

Another category of evidence gaps not assessed by the USPSTF analytic framework involves the D&I of a preventive service once it has been recommended. The USPSTF does not routinely consider gaps related to D&I, but the committee agreed it was crucial to include as part of a taxonomy of clinical prevention evidence gaps. How a preventive service affects morbidity and mortality is necessary but insufficient for effective clinical prevention practice—preventive services must also be feasible, scalable, and sustainable for clinicians to implement and for patients to adhere to.

As described in more detail in the following sections, the committee decided on a taxonomy consisting of two sections: (1) three different facets of prevention-related evidence gaps: foundational issues, analytic framework gaps, and D&I gaps; and (2) two facets for use in outlining a research agenda. With this general structure, the committee assessed specific facets by applying them to existing I statements and evaluating how they were able to characterize the evidence gaps described in those statements. This process was carried out on approximately a dozen different I statements, with the taxonomy being fine-tuned according to the lessons learned from each exercise.

In addition to developing the taxonomy, the committee thought it was also important to offer some direction for how the taxonomy could be used by the USPSTF and other clinical practice guideline developers. As described in the next section, the committee members developed a workflow to outline the identification of evidence gaps and development of a research agenda.

WORKFLOW

The committee agreed early on that it would be crucial to describe both its taxonomy and the way that taxonomy should be applied to maximize its utility. The committee did this by developing a workflow graphic to visualize the appropriate steps in using the taxonomy to characterize evidence gaps, prioritize those gaps, and describe the type of research necessary to close the gaps (see Figure 4-5 for the overall workflow). This section describes the workflow, which can be viewed as a companion guide on how to use the taxonomy, along with its purpose and how it may be used.

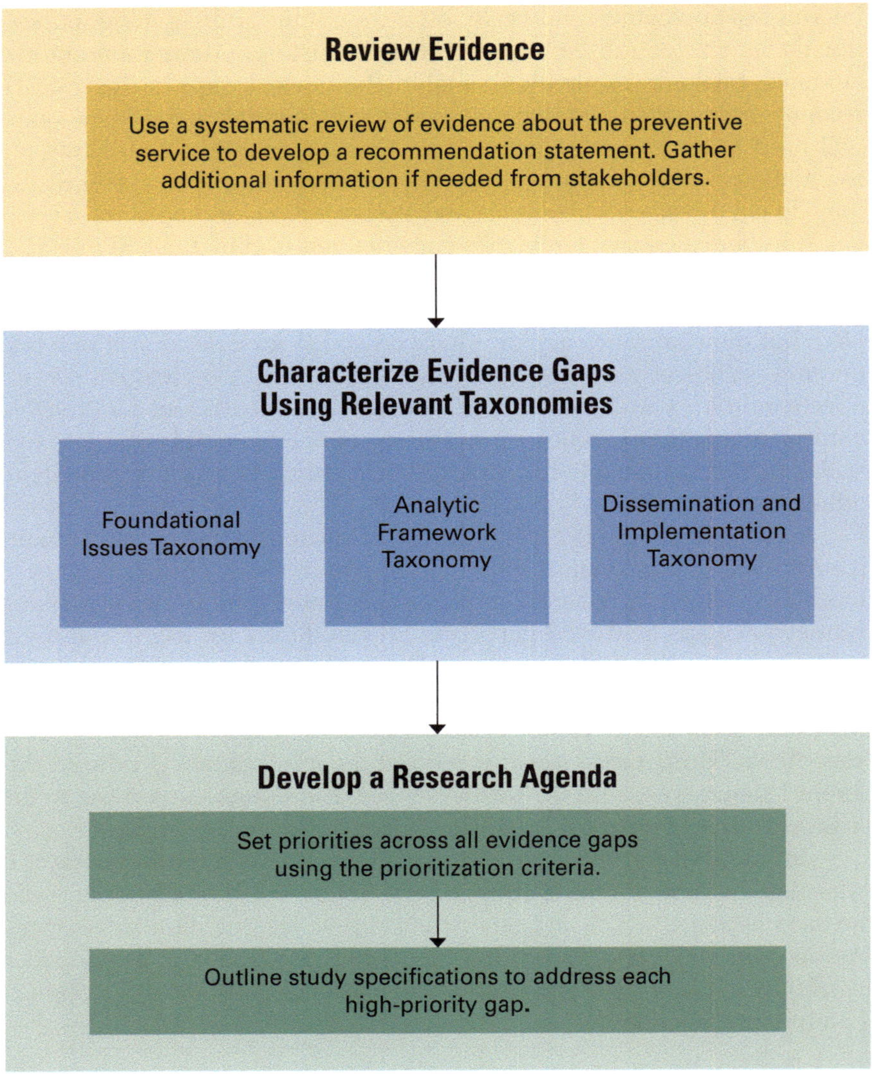

FIGURE 4-5 The workflow for identifying evidence gaps in clinical prevention with the taxonomy.
NOTE: To view the taxonomy as an interactive graphic, see https://www.nap.edu/resource/26351.

The first step is to review the evidence concerning a particular preventive service in order to develop a recommendation statement. As far as this applies to the USPSTF, this would be after they receive their draft evidence review from an Evidence-based Practice Center with which they have contracted for the review. However, the workflow does not assume its only users will be members of the USPSTF; and any interested party may carry out the review of evidence. In some cases, it will be necessary to gather additional information from stakeholders to outline issues around D&I.

Once the review of evidence has been completed, the next step is to use the taxonomy (as described in the next section) to identify the gaps that exist in the evidence. These gaps will be placed in one of three facets of the taxonomy: foundational, analytic framework, and D&I. Most evidence gaps that would lead to an I statement will primarily characterize foundational and/or analytic framework gaps; that is, those evidence gaps that have traditionally been considered by the USPSTF. However, the committee recognizes that gaps in D&I evidence are also important to address to improve health outcomes related to clinical preventive services. Thus, although it was not mentioned in the statement of task, the committee chose to make D&I part of its taxonomy.

Once the three types of evidence gaps have been identified and characterized with the taxonomy, the next step in the workflow is to develop a research agenda. The first step in this process is to prioritize the various gaps. This is done using prioritization criteria, as discussed in the next section. The goal is to get a clear idea of which evidence gaps make sense to address first, so that finite resources for prevention research can be put to optimal use.

With a list of prioritized evidence gaps, the final step is to outline the key research studies needed to address the high-priority evidence gaps. The necessary studies are specified according to a set of characteristics that are an extension of the PICOTS framework.

Not every interested party will necessarily carry out every step in the workflow. Some users may choose to focus on the traditional USPSTF concerns and apply only the first two parts of the taxonomy—covering foundational issues and analytic framework issues—and not address D&I. Others, such as funders, might focus on evidence gaps identified by the USPSTF or another guideline-making group and prioritize the gaps differently than the USPSTF might to develop a research agenda that reflects the highest-priority research needs based on their assessment. The committee envisions that the results of the prioritization step may vary depending on the relative weights different groups or individuals place on the criteria evaluated, which in turn could result in different research needs receiving the highest priority among different stakeholders. For example, some funders may prioritize promoting health equity and addressing health disparities in clinical prevention, thus focusing on research needs that have identified populations that experience health disparities. Ultimately, the taxonomy and workflow will ensure that stakeholders invested in clinical prevention research will share a language to advance the field.

TAXONOMY FOR CLASSIFYING EVIDENCE GAPS

As already described, in developing its taxonomy for classifying evidence gaps the committee chose to modify the analytic framework used by the USPSTF to describe evidence gaps. This section comprises the first three facets of the taxonomy: foundational issues, analytic framework gaps, and D&I gaps. The result is an approach that has significant overlap with the USPSTF methodology in assessing linkages between preventive services and health outcomes but expands its considerations of evidence gaps beyond those directly related to the analytic framework.

The taxonomy provides a systematic way of describing evidence gaps with a clear list of categories and a controlled vocabulary for consistency across evidence reviews. Furthermore, by offering a list of the different classes of evidence gaps that may play a role in analyzing a preventive service, the taxonomy and the workflow offer a road map for researchers and funders. The formal listing of categories also makes it easier to compare the evidence gaps among different preventive services and, ultimately, to prioritize the gaps and specify the research needed to address them (see Box 4-1 for a comprehensive view of the five facets of the evidence gaps taxonomy).

While many evidence gaps noted in the USPSTF recommendations refer to linkages in the analytic framework, some evidence gaps did refer to foundational issues. Foundational issues include gaps in a basic understanding of disease processes, psychometric properties of a service, and whether any preventive service exists. Accordingly, the committee created a "foundational issues" facet. Not every I statement will have foundational issues to address, but they will be important in some cases as prerequisites or complements to address analytic framework questions.

The third facet of the evidence gaps taxonomy is D&I, which covers an aspect of preventive services that the USPSTF traditionally does not address in recommendation statements. However, identifying and understanding evidence gaps related to D&I are important aspects of improving preventive services and should be included in any framework aimed at developing a research agenda for such services.

BOX 4-1
Clinical Prevention Evidence Gaps Taxonomy Terms

- Evidence Gaps Taxonomy
  - Foundational Issues
    - Condition Definition and Nomenclature
    - Disease Processes
    - Preventive Services
    - Development of Standards
    - Psychometric Properties
  - Analytic Framework
    - Risk Assessment and Health Equity Considerations
      - Behavioral and Sociodemographic Risk Factors
        - Country of Origin
        - Ethnicity
        - Gender
        - Race
        - Sexual Orientation
        - Socioeconomic Position
      - Biological and Clinical Risk Factors
        - Age
        - Comorbidities
        - Family History
        - Genetics and Molecular Biomarkers
        - Pregnancy Status
        - Sex (as a biological variable)
    - Early Detection
      - Early Detection
    - Intermediate Outcomes
      - Effects of Treatment on Intermediate Outcomes
      - Association of Intermediate Outcomes with Morbidity and Mortality
    - Effectiveness
      - Effects of Screening on Morbidity and Mortality
      - Effects of Treatment (behavioral intervention or preventive medication) on Morbidity and Mortality
    - Harms
      - Screening Harms
      - Treatment Harms
  - Dissemination and Implementation
    - Size
    - Scope of Services, Including Costs
    - Scalability
    - Sustainability
    - Penetration of Program into the Intended Audience
    - Implementation of the Scope of Services
    - Participation in the Program
    - Effectiveness of the Program

continued

BOX 4-1 Continued

- Research Agenda Taxonomy
  - Prioritization Criteria
    - Population Impact
    - Equity
    - Centrality
    - Relative Importance
    - Time Urgency
    - Adoptability
    - Value, Including Economic Considerations
    - Feasibility of Research
  - Study Specifications
    - Population
    - Intervention
    - Comparison Group
    - Outcome(s)
    - Timeframe for Follow-Up
    - Setting
    - Aggregability
    - Design Considerations
    - Potential Funders and Mechanisms

Foundational Gaps

The existence of some foundational evidence gaps may mean guideline developers are not able to continue assessing a preventive service. Foundational evidence gaps seem likely to affect the magnitude of certainty regarding harms and benefits if they are to affect a recommendation or I statement at all. However, the USPSTF recommendations and I statements included enough reference to the following categories that the committee felt it necessary to identify a separate taxonomy facet. The committee developed the following categories for foundational evidence gaps related to clinical preventive services (see Figure 4-6 for the corresponding workflow section).

Condition Definition and Nomenclature

It is vital that researchers and clinicians working in a particular area agree on the meanings of the terms they use to describe the condition, disease, screening, intervention, results, and so forth. Having a precise definition of the disease or condition under consideration is particularly important, as it helps ensure that study findings can be compared,

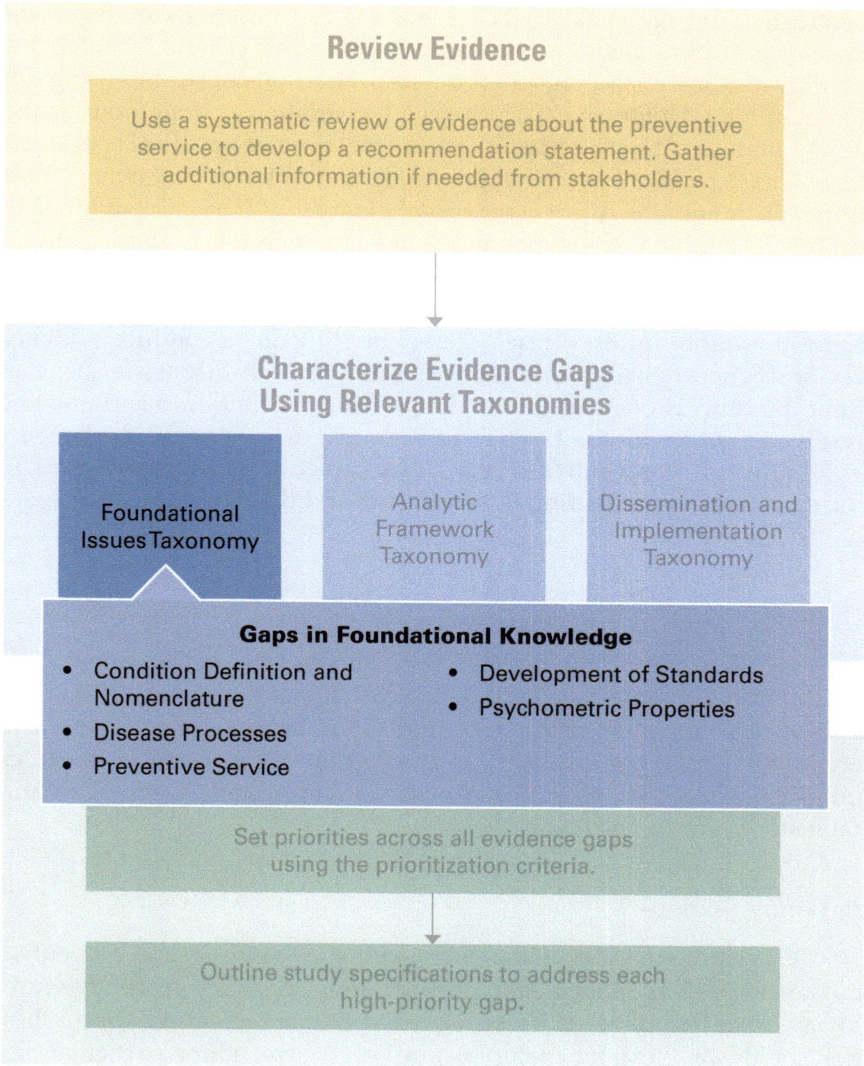

FIGURE 4-6 The workflow with foundational evidence gaps facet.

contrasted, and aggregated. This is not to say that variations in a diagnosis create a gap, but rather that variations in diagnostic criteria can affect the validity of research findings that combine the results of studies using different criteria. Unfortunately, there can be variation in definitions across a field for a variety of reasons. For example, different medical specialties have varying definitions of hypertension, and different researchers have different definitions of myalgic encephalomyelitis/chronic fatigue syndrome. In addition, some diagnoses, like attention deficit/hyperactivity disorder, have changed over time, making it difficult to compare studies. In some cases, it can be difficult to know if two reports are discussing the same condition. In other cases, it may be difficult to conduct evidence reviews when not all terminology is known. Such inconsistencies can limit the conclusions that can be drawn from the literature and must be resolved in order for the USPSTF to comprehensively assess the benefits and harms of a preventive service. This category encompasses gaps in the evidence base regarding nomenclature and the definition of diseases or conditions.

Disease Processes

Are there important details about the causes, development, and results of the disease that remain unclear? If so, it can make it difficult to determine the most effective methods of screening, for instance, or to accurately gauge the effects of an intervention. This category includes unresolved issues related to the disease's pathophysiology, etiology, natural history, and comorbidities.

Preventive Services

"Preventive services" refers to screening, counseling, and preventive medication—three strategies of primary and secondary preventive care. There can be foundational issues related to each of these three approaches. It is not always clear, for example, how best to screen for a particular disease. For example, the recommendation for colorectal cancer screenings refers to multiple types of screening tests. To be recommended by the USPSTF, a screening test should be consistent and well defined. Foundational evidence gaps regarding preventive services may include what devices or technology may be required to administer it, how frequently it should be administered, or if it has any method issues (e.g., does this test require a special diet?).

Development of Standards

Standards play a vital role in medical science as an agreed-upon set of rules for how data are collected, procedures are conducted, decisions are made, and so forth. Most research protocols offer detailed standards on how to perform a screening. For example, for occult blood screening of colorectal cancer, research protocols detail dietary restrictions, timing of collection, and so on. Inconsistent research standards between studies can affect the validity of research findings that combine results of studies using different standards, thus creating a gap. In that sense, the need for clear standards is similar to the need for standardized nomenclature and disease definitions—both help provide a solid foundation for everything else. In some cases, what seems to be conflicting evidence regarding a particular preventive service or intervention may actually be an indication of a lack of standards in the performance of the service or in the measurement of the outcome, and it may be necessary to clear up these inconsistencies before a clear conclusion can be drawn about the effectiveness of the service.

Psychometric Properties

"Psychometric properties" refers to reliability and validity of a measurement tool (Asunta et al., 2019). Once a tool is identified and its use has been standardized, the tool itself will also require assessment as to its sensitivity, specificity, predictive value, reliability, and other factors. While there is an argument that these issues belong in the Analytic Framework, the committee feels these are foundational issues that affect test performance, which will be demonstrated (or not) in the Analytic Framework. Without evidence of rigorous evaluation, the USPSTF is unlikely to weigh in on recommending a service. For example, the USPSTF reviewed "risk assessment instruments used to identify children for whom preventive interventions might be indicated and found limited and inconsistent evidence on the validity and reliability of these tools," which served as a contributing factor to the topic's I statement (USPSTF, 2018b).

Other

There may be foundational evidence gaps that do not clearly fit into any of the previous categories. The committee envisions that those who manage the taxonomy will update it as appropriate. Because of this, it is probable that subject matter not currently in the taxonomy but that is consistently added would eventually be developed into its own category within its respective facet. This applies to all facets of the taxonomy.

Analytic Framework Gaps

The committee first identified evidence gaps that can be observed in the context of the USPSTF's generic analytic framework. Most of those gaps are associated with links between an action (i.e., screening, behavioral interventions, preventive medication) and an outcome (e.g., early detection of a condition, adverse effects associated with screening or treatment, reduced morbidity and mortality). These questions include "Does screening leading to early detection?" and "Does screening lead to adverse effects?" Because the analytic framework anchors their assessment of a preventive service, most evidence gaps identified by the USPSTF are gaps in these actions, outcomes, or the linkages between them. The committee classified these evidence gaps according to the outcomes shown in the USPSTF's analytic frameworks: Risk Assessment and Health Equity Considerations, Early Detection, Intermediate Outcomes, Effectiveness, and Harms. Those five categories form the first level of the committee's analytic framework taxonomy, with various subcategories included within each main category (see Figure 4-7 for the corresponding workflow section).

Risk Assessment and Health Equity Considerations

In the typical analytic framework produced by the USPSTF as exemplified by Figures 4-1 and 4-2, risk assessment serves as the beginning of the process in which a clinician offers or does not offer a preventive service to a patient. In some cases, the USPSTF recommends that clinicians offer a preventive service to the entire adult population at risk of acquiring a disease, such as screening for depression in adults, screening for hypertension, or screening for unhealthy drug use (USPSTF, 2016b, 2020b, 2021a).

However, most of the topics assessed by the USPSTF require a clinician to perform some kind of risk assessment as to whether the risk or burden of disease may be higher for an individual based on a number of risk factors. For example, a clinician may offer a nonpregnant patient a combination of behavioral counseling and pharmacotherapy after they confirm that the patient uses tobacco (USPSTF, 2021e). A clinician would also assess behavioral risk factors, asking about sexual activity and injection drug use before suggesting a patient take PrEP to prevent acquisition of HIV (USPSTF, 2019).

Many evidence gaps identified by the USPSTF in published recommendation or I statements include the lack of information about the way a disease or a preventive service affects specific subpopulations. Another

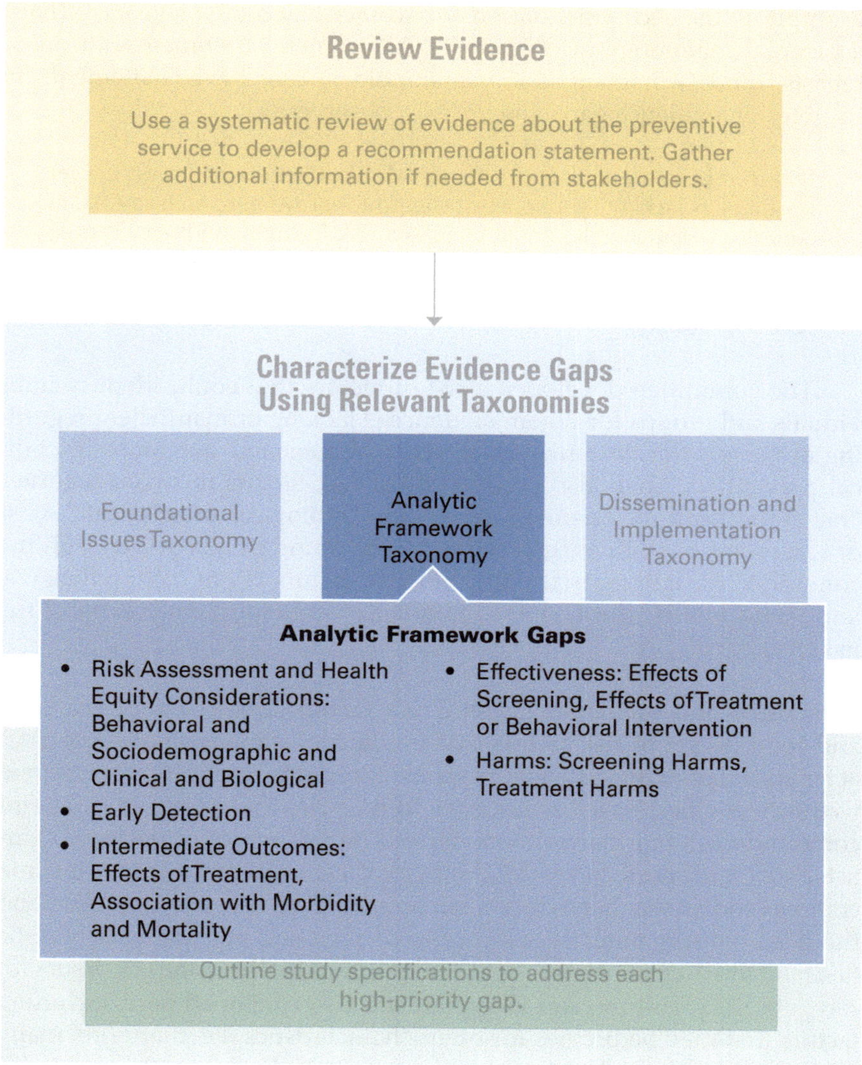

FIGURE 4-7 The workflow with analytic framework evidence gaps facet.

example is the recommendation for women aged 50–74 years to have a biennial mammogram (B grade). "All women," "women with dense breasts," and "women aged 75 years or older" each have I statements. In its notes on evidence gaps, the USPSTF observes:

> Direct evidence about any differential effectiveness of breast cancer screening is lacking for important subgroups of women, such as African American women, who are at increased risk for dying of breast cancer, and older women, for whom balancing the potential benefits and harms of screening may become increasingly challenging with advancing age. (USPSTF, 2016a)

The committee developed a list of factors that could identify individuals and groups for whom evidence is lacking or insufficient regarding any aspect of the linkages between actions and outcomes in clinical prevention. They also grouped most risk factors in two categories, "behavioral and sociodemographic," and "biological and clinical." A list of important respective risk factors can be found in Box 4-1, though the committee recognizes that the list of risk factors is not comprehensive, and AHRQ, NIH, the USPSTF, or other stakeholders may expand the list as needed.

Behavioral and sociodemographic risk factors This category is a large and complex set of risk factors that encompasses many of the risk characteristics that, with sufficient research, can guide application of preventive services. Some factors are easy to measure and verify (e.g., age or comorbidities), but many others depend on self-report of personal characteristics and social exposures. Many risk factors in this category include complex individual behaviors, such as substance use, exercise, diet, and the behavioral manifestations of mental illnesses, and patients may be hesitant to disclose some social circumstances. The complex issues of race, ethnicity, culture, and inequality are also contained here, including factors that may be proxies for other characteristics. Furthermore, many behavioral and sociodemographic characteristics have genetic, metabolic, and other biological underpinnings, and the pathways from genotype to phenotype are often not fully understood (Lappalainen and MacArthur, 2021) or malleable.

Sociodemographic risk factors may also serve as a surrogate for social determinants of health, which are the "social and economic conditions" and "fundamental drivers of those conditions" in which communities live, rather than the immediate needs of any one individual (Castrucci and Auerbach, 2019; CSDH, 2008; Davidson et al., 2020, 2021).

Biological and clinical risk factors Many risk factors that underpin preventive interventions are explicitly "biological" and are often primarily assessed measuring genetic, metabolic, physiological, or other biomarkers, such as polygenic risk scores, blood pressure, and plasma total cholesterol levels or imaging outcomes. However, despite many successes, all biomarkers have measurement issues that may challenge risk assessment and limit application. Also, importantly, many persons who are otherwise generally suitable for a preventive intervention may have comorbid conditions of varying import or severity that may substantially alter the evidence base for that suitability, such as diseases that modify metabolic risk (e.g., diabetes) or personal behaviors (e.g., obsessive-compulsive disorder or eating disorders). Various treatments of comorbid conditions may also change target disease detection or progression (e.g., radiation-induced myocarditis from cancer treatment or weight gain from anti-psychotic drugs).

Early Detection

"Early detection" and the related evidence gaps refers to any problem in disease screening in which a disease or condition that appears to be earlier in its natural course can be detected, but when the condition is followed into the future, the untoward clinical outcomes are the same or worse, even when considering the total amount of time the disease has been in place. A useful example is that some colon tumors may be detected that seem to be in earlier stages (i.e., they are smaller and less dysplastic, but still may have the same disease and mortality outcomes over a common follow-p interval). This has often been referred to as "lead-time bias" or "length-time bias" (MacDonald et al., 2011). Here, research studies must better understand whether "early detection" and management of a disease actually favorably alter the longer-term clinical outcomes, to justify the preventive service.

Intermediate Outcomes

The intermediary outcomes category comprises evidence gaps in "pathologic, physiologic, psychologic, social, or behavioral measures related to a preventive intervention" that are "not [health outcomes] in and of themselves" (Wolff et al., 2018, p. S5). For example, an intermediate outcome is the change in blood pressure. Due to the proximal pathophysiology between blood pressure and morbidity and mortality outcomes, an evidence base linking regular blood pressure screenings (preventive service) with lower blood pressure (intermediate outcome) may be strongly considered by the USPSTF in the absence of sufficient evidence linking blood pressure screenings directly with morbidity and mortality outcomes. While the USPSTF "exercises caution when making a recommendation that depends in large part on the evidence linking [intermediate outcomes] and [health outcomes]," addressing gaps in intermediate outcomes may still help strengthen the evidence base for or against a preventive service (Wolff et al., 2018, p. S7).

The committee envisions two main subcategories in the intermediate outcomes category, although (as with the other categories) those using the taxonomy will likely find others that fit in this category as well. The following are two subcategories of evidence gaps:

- The effects of treatment, including behavioral interventions (i.e., does the treatment or behavioral intervention affect intermediate outcomes?)
- Association with morbidity and mortality (i.e., are the intermediate outcomes linked with health outcomes?)

In the blood pressure example, the first category would include questions about whether a particular treatment—such as a low sodium diet or the use of an ACE (angiotensin-converting enzyme) inhibitor—leads to lower blood pressure, while the second category would contain questions such as whether lowering an individual's blood pressure as a result of treatment leads to a longer life expectancy or lowers the risk of stroke.

Effectiveness

The effectiveness category involves questions relating to whether an early preventive service (i.e., screening, behavioral counseling, or medication) is either effective in decreasing morbidity or mortality or, in the absence of such data, intermediate outcomes (Wolff et al., 2018). Evidence gaps in this category will involve situations in which there are insufficient data to conclude that a preventive service is effective.

Harms

The harms category includes evidence gaps related to whether the preventive intervention or the treatment leads to adverse effects. As with the effectiveness category, there are two main subcategories:

- Harms associated with the screening or assessment
- Harms associated with the treatment

Evidence gaps in this category will involve situations in which there are insufficient data to conclude that a preventive intervention or a treatment leads to harms. In some cases, the USPSTF or other guideline developers may note that there are evidence gaps regarding harms of a preventive service, but ultimately not prioritize research addressing them.

Dissemination and Implementation Gaps

Historically, the USPSTF has not reviewed issues of D&I in its recommendation statements, focusing instead on whether sufficient evidence exists to conclude that a particular preventive service is effective in reducing harms. If this is the sole focus, then the taxonomy would be complete with just the two previous facets—the foundational taxonomy and the analytic framework taxonomy. However, the committee chose to approach the taxonomy from a more holistic point of view, recognizing that there is more to the decision of which preventive services to encourage than simply determining which ones have the most supporting evidence. As D&I each have multiple definitions, different guideline developers may choose to assess the dissemination of their own guidelines, the implementation of the preventive services, or a combination of the two. The committee notes that in a recent publication, USPSTF members and AHRQ staff wrote the following:

> Although the use of implementation research is not within the scope of the USPSTF's deliberations, it notes that there are critical questions about how to best implement recommended clinical preventive services in primary care practices. Additional implementation and translational research will increase the value of the USPSTF's work and would be helpful in its deliberations. (Mabry-Hernandez et al., 2018, p. S98)

The authors do not elaborate on how such information would be helpful.

In particular, the success of a preventive service depends not only on its effectiveness in a research setting but also on how well it can be disseminated and implemented. If an intervention is difficult to disseminate or impractical to implement, it may not be a good choice as a preventive service. Consider, for example, computed tomography (CT) angiography, which can create detailed scans of blood vessels. While it is certainly a useful diagnostic tool, it is expensive, and thus there are questions concerning how widely CT angiography is likely to be used in preventive services, even in cases where it may help decrease morbidity or mortality in a group of at-risk individuals. Additionally, implementation is a major factor in terms of health equity and access.

To categorize evidence gaps related to D&I, the committee chose an existing framework developed to design and evaluate health promotion or disease prevention programs, referred to as 4S/PIPE (Äikäs et al., 2017, 2019, 2020; Pronk, 2003). The 4S component refers to four elements of designing a health promotion program: size, scope, scalability, and sustainability. By contrast, PIPE is an impact metric with four different components: penetration, implementation, participation, and effectiveness. Feedback loops are included in the model that connect 4S to PIPE in an effort to ensure that insights and learnings from the PIPE component continue to inform design features that are part of the 4S component. Together they provide a breakdown of important components of the design, dissemination, and implementation of a program, so that evidence gaps related to D&I can generally be placed into one of the eight slots defined by 4S/PIPE (see Figure 4-8 for the corresponding workflow section).

Size

"Size" refers to the magnitude, extent, relative aggregate amount or number, or dose of the program or intervention that has an impact on the user, thereby creating the desired effect (i.e., effect size). The size of an intervention can refer to a variety of aspects, depending on the details of the intervention, but it always refers to the magnitude, amount, or dose of whatever is being done or the amount of change that is generated. Thus, for a particular implementation of a preventive intervention, size might refer to the number of individuals or patients who would be targeted, the number of clinicians or health care workers who would be involved, the intervention dose or amount of change effort that is presented as part of the intervention, or the amount of change that is generated at an individual patient level or the group level of participating individuals. A size-related D&I evidence gap might be an uncertainty in the number of practitioners who would be competent to implement an intervention, the number of individuals who should be targeted, or the amount of change anticipated in a certain subpopulation. From an equity perspective, research results that provide an estimate of the effect size that may be anticipated when a certain preventive intervention or screening is implemented may not be applicable to specific subpopulations. Biases that providers or researchers may have in screenings or counseling processes can contribute to an evidence-generation problem that manifests itself in the effect size of the intervention. At the same time, anticipated effect sizes may not be achieved when implementation approaches for certain subgroups are not commensurate with their needs, thereby generating unequal impacts across various subpopulations.

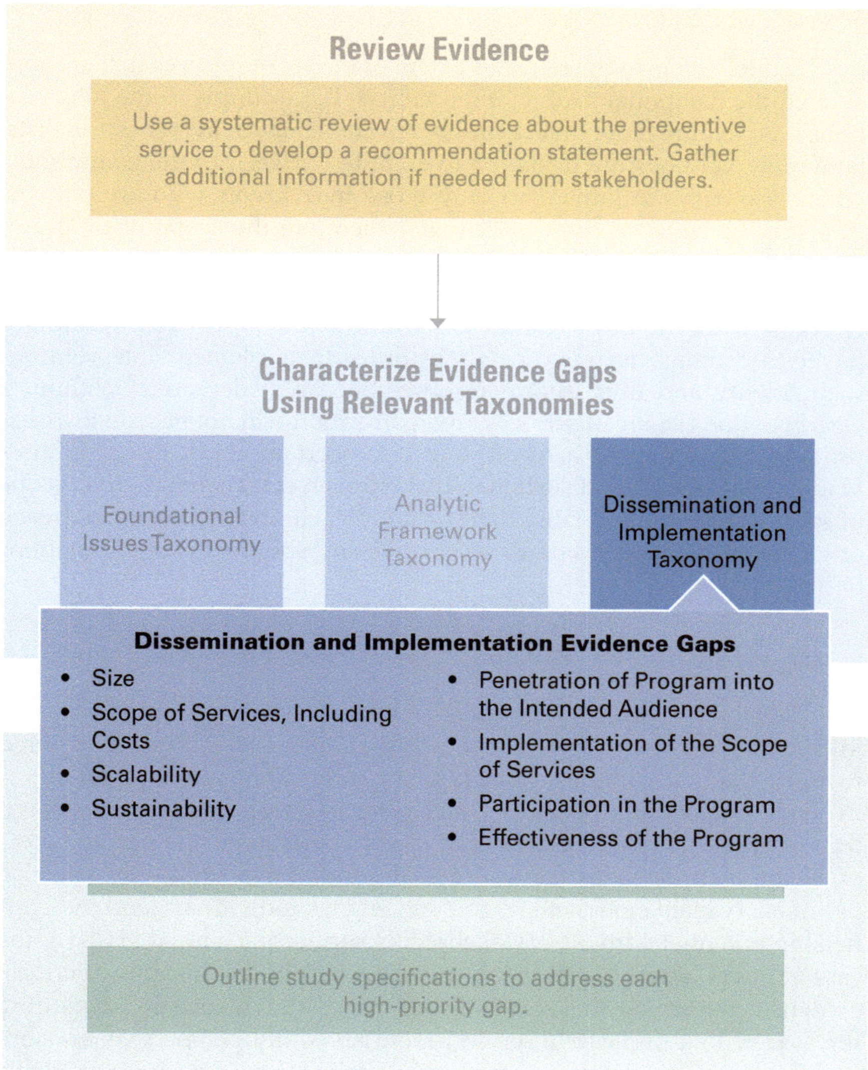

FIGURE 4-8 The workflow with dissemination and implementation evidence gaps facet.

Scope of Services, Including Cost

"Scope" refers to the range or extent of the set of services that are considered the components of an intervention. For example, some interventions may require more time, a number of clinicians, or involve specialists. Some interventions are designed to include outreach to the community, whereas others are limited to only those individuals who are patients of a specific clinic or care system, and therefore the scope of programmatic aspects and services will differ. Another important consideration is that the scope of program services is directly related to program costs. An understanding of program costs would allow a provider, vendor, or payer to estimate resource needs in order to implement interventions with fidelity and thus inform resource allocation decisions. Without a clearly defined scope of services an organization will not be able to assess program costs and, as a result, will be uncertain about the program's viability, scalability, and sustainability. From an equity perspective, scope of services is directly related to, for example, culturally specific outreach or inclusion of strategies that are sensitive and specific to subpopulations of interest.

Scalability

"Scalability" refers to how easily an intervention can be spread from an initial small number of practitioners to the much larger number required to make the intervention available to an entire population. Scalability is dependent upon multiple factors, including, but not limited to, the willingness of members of the target population to participate, the per-unit costs of the intervention in the context of total resource availability, the effective use of all available media to recruit and engage individuals, and the partnership potential with other stakeholders supporting similar goals. In the case of novel interventions, there may be a lack of key insights or critical evidence concerning this scalability, creating an evidence gap regarding the D&I of that preventive service. From an equity perspective, scalability of a preventive intervention may be hindered by data from available research results that are limited to observations representative of a single population (e.g., only white Caucasian males), whereas gaps exist among specific target populations (e.g., non-white female populations).

Sustainability

"Sustainability" refers to how easy it will be to maintain a program once it has reached the full necessary extent to cover a population. This in turn will depend on such factors as to whether there is institutional buy-in and sources of funding that can be relied on over the long term. More specifically, it refers to the long-term, ongoing support for the program in relation to an accepted value proposition that balances allocated resources (e.g., time, money, people, or other available means) against generated revenues or benefits and includes the confirmation of long-term program support through adequate proof of performance. As with scalability, it may be difficult to judge the likely sustainability of a novel intervention that is significantly different from existing interventions. From an equity perspective, preventive interventions that are sustained over time should generate outcomes that are equally distributed across various subpopulations. Evaluations of programs implemented in the "real world" are critical to provide such insights, and such evaluations may be designed using the PIPE Impact Metric yet to be discussed. Evaluation outcomes in this regard are to be fed back into the 4S design cycle in order to improve program design and generate improvements in outcomes.

Penetration of the Program into the Intended Audience

A measure of how widely disseminated and implemented an intervention is, "penetration" refers to the percentage of the target audience that is reached by the intervention—that is, the percentage that is made aware of the intervention and to whom it is available. For new interventions with novel characteristics it may be difficult to gauge the likely penetration—thus the need for studies of penetration and the existence of evidence gaps when such studies have not be carried out. From an equity perspective, outreach to subpopulations needs to be coordinated in a way that resonates with such audiences, be culturally appropriate, and use media that ensure all members of the audience may be reached.

Implementation of the Scope of Services

Implementation is a measure of the extent to which an intervention is being carried out in accordance with the standardized set of guidelines developed for that intervention or the specific work plan associated with the service. The interpretation of the X rays or CT images used in screening can be complex, for instance, with great variation in the interpretation among practitioners; such variation could blunt the effectiveness of a preventive service that would otherwise be quite valuable. Alternatively, outreach efforts related to mammography screening may use a variety of strategies in order to achieve a certain performance target; not achieving the target may be related to incomplete implementation of the work plans specific to such strategies. Thus, evidence gaps concerning the implementation of an intervention could make it difficult to judge how effectively the intervention could be applied across an entire population.

From an equity perspective, it is critical that strategies designed to close disparity gaps are fully implemented according to plan. Failure to do so will undoubtedly generate suboptimal outcomes.

Participation in the Program

Participation refers to the uptake of a preventive service by individuals to whom the service has been offered. While penetration is concerned with the percentage of the target population that is reached by the intervention, participation examines that part of the population and asks how many of them actually do take advantage of the opportunity. Together, penetration and participation indicate the percentage of the total target audience who have the intervention available and take advantage of it. Participation depends on a wide variety of factors, including how well practitioners explain the purpose of the intervention and its value. Participation rates are also likely to vary by population characteristics—race and socioeconomic position, for instance. While there are broad patterns visible in the data on participation rates that make it possible to guess what the participation in a new type of intervention is likely to be, there will always be a great deal of uncertainty concerning the actual rates until the relevant studies have been carried out. Thus, evidence gaps are likely for this category for any new type of preventive service. From an equity perspective, participation in preventive interventions may be closely related to the degree of outreach and attention provided to the target audience. For example, despite awareness of the availability of infectious disease vaccines, subpopulations may be hesitant to engage and participate for various reasons, including lack of trust in the health care system. For such specific subpopulations additional strategies to overcome vaccine hesitancy are needed to close the gaps in vaccine rates.

Effectiveness of the Program

The last category, effectiveness, examines the portion of a target population that has participated in an intervention and asks in how many of those the intervention was effective in terms of reducing morbidity or mortality or according to some other desired endpoint. Measuring effectiveness can be challenging, particularly since it can be difficult to know on an individual level what the outcome would have been without the intervention and because many of the desired endpoints, such as mortality and various morbidities, may not become apparent for years or even decades after the intervention. Many studies of effectiveness may depend on measures of intermediate outcomes. Depending on the intervention and the desired outcome, there may be a number of types of evidence gaps related to its effectiveness. Effectiveness may be considered as the proportion of "successes" generated—how many people among those who participated achieved a successful outcome? From an equity perspective, the proportion of successful interventions among the members of the subpopulation can be directly compared to other subpopulations, may be considered in the context of the 4Ss of program design, and may inform potential changes to be made in future implementation efforts.

The committee emphasizes that the D&I evidence gap taxonomy described here is not intended as a finished product but rather as a starting point for a taxonomy that is more closely tailored to the evidence gaps most likely to appear related to the D&I of preventive interventions. The committee settled on 4S/PIPE as a well-established framework that has clear application to the D&I of preventive services because it wished to offer a concrete example that would demonstrate the value of including D&I in the overall taxonomy, but the committee members believe that more suitable terms might be developed by others.

The committee recognizes that, unlike the case with the foundational and analytic framework facets, the D&I facet requires the USPSTF to cover new ground, as it has generally not included any dissemination or implementation issues as in its statements, except under "Considerations for Practice." However, the committee members believe that the USPSTF members are likely to have experience in the area that will allow them to identify various evidence gaps related to D&I, particularly if they use the committee's taxonomy as a guide. To the extent that the USPSTF members do not have the capacity or expertise to identify these gaps, they might contract with outside experts to conduct evidence reviews and do so (see Chapter 5 for more detail). However it is done, the committee believes it is important that the USPSTF and other groups invested in improving clinical prevention research identify evidence gaps related to the D&I of the preventive services. This is particularly true when it comes to the potential for D&I to address gaps in health equity.

Crosscutting Issues

While the committee divided the various issues related to recommending preventive services into three facets—foundational, analytic framework, and D&I—for the purpose of creating a taxonomy of these issues, it recognizes that in the real world the division is not nearly as neat as the taxonomy might seem to indicate. In reality, there is a great deal of overlap and interaction among these three broad categories. Foundational gaps in knowledge about the pathophysiology of a disease are likely to result in various gaps in knowledge related to the true effectiveness of screening, for instance, and advances in foundational knowledge could lead to modifications in screening or even completely new techniques. Indeed, the close interplay between foundational issues and analytic framework issues means that there is a significant gray area between the two where it is not always clear whether an issue should be considered foundational or part of the analytic framework. There can be similar interplay between foundational issues and D&I or between the analytic framework and D&I.

Thus, it is important to keep in mind when categorizing the various evidence gaps related to a preventive intervention that various crosscutting issues can arise, and each of these must be dealt with on a case-by-case basis as there is no easy way to account for them in the taxonomy as defined.

TAXONOMY FOR DEVELOPING THE RESEARCH AGENDA

Once a set of evidence gaps has been classified according to the elements of the taxonomy, the next step in the process is to develop a research agenda to address those gaps. As envisioned by the committee, putting together such a research agenda will involve two steps: prioritizing the various evidence gaps and then specifying the type of research that will be required to fill each gap—or at least each of the high-priority evidence gaps. These two steps use two respective facets that complement the rest of the taxonomy of evidence gaps in clinical research. The end result of this process will be a collection of prioritized research needs, with studies outlined to address each research need.

Prioritizing the Evidence Gaps

One of the key purposes of the taxonomy is to make it possible to characterize the various evidence gaps in a consistent way that allows researchers and policy makers to compare the evidence gaps and to prioritize them. This prioritization facet (along with the study specification facet, described next) differs from the first three facets of the taxonomy because it involves value judgments. The facets that categorize evidence gaps serve as the traditional elements of a taxonomy, for systematic categorization. For example, for a topic like screening for autism spectrum disorder (ASD) among asymptomatic children aged 18–30 months, it would be expected that multiple parties with different interests would consistently identify evidence gaps within the analytic framework facet. However, researchers and funders may have different areas of interest in addressing any or all of those gaps and thus may prioritize them differently. The prioritization facet offers consistent language on which to base those judgments (see Figure 4-9 for the corresponding workflow section).

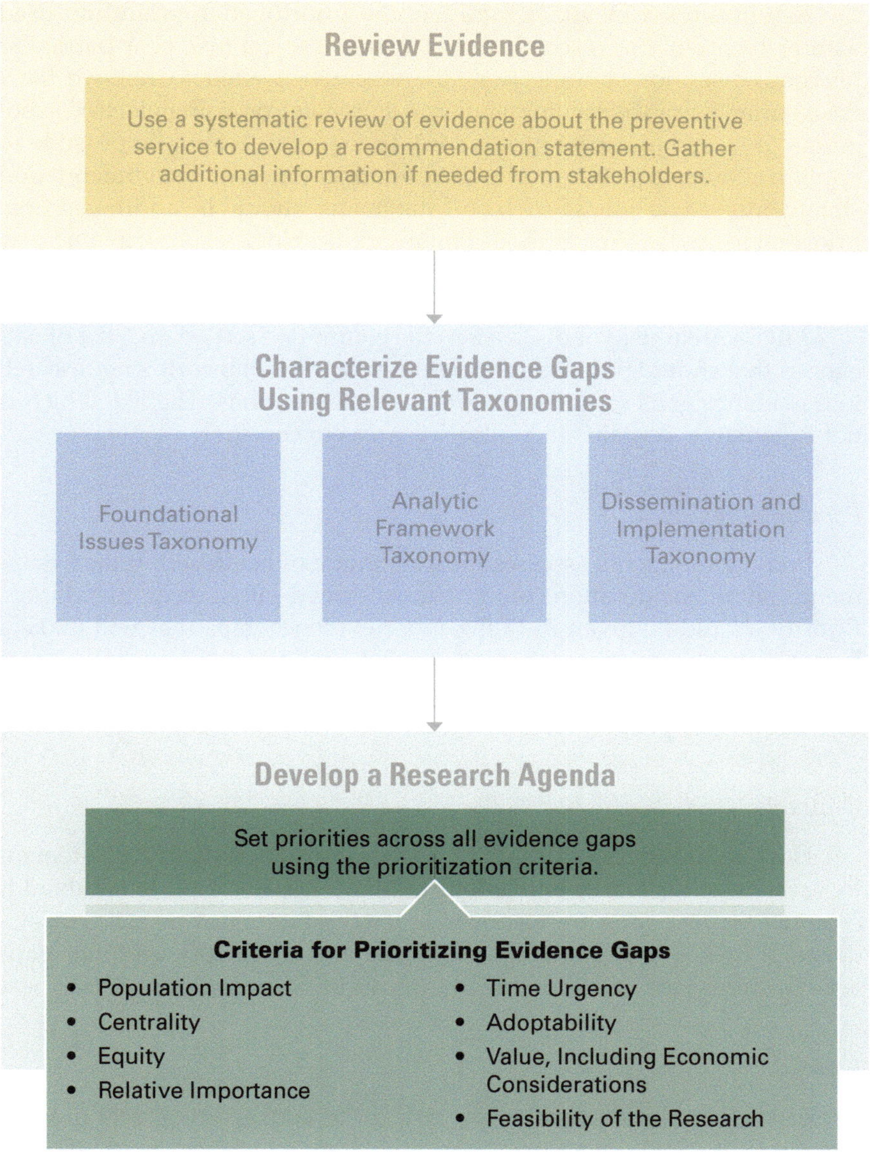

FIGURE 4-9 The workflow with prioritization criteria facet.

As envisioned by the committee, the prioritization would be used mainly to order the research needs within the context of a particular preventive service or topic (e.g., the research needed to remove the I designation from the recommendation statement on using electrocardiograms to screen for atrial fibrillation). In theory, it would be possible to apply a similar process to prioritize among different recommendation statements—to decide, say, which I statements should be addressed first. Prioritizing evidence gaps should follow clinical logic as well; a topic may remain an I statement because the body of evidence required to recommend against the service (D grade) may be too large to be feasible.

After a great deal of discussion, the committee settled on a list of categories that should be taken into consideration when prioritizing research into evidence gaps related to preventive interventions. The list, which is not exhaustive, contains the following areas to consider:

Population Impact

Population impact assesses the magnitude of net benefit if the I statement under consideration could be transformed into a recommendation. Priority should be given to filling those evidence gaps that will make a larger difference in people's lives or that will affect significantly more people, rather than to filling those gaps where the effect will be smaller or where fewer people will be affected.

Centrality

How important is a particular evidence gap to updating an I statement to a recommendation or one letter grade recommendation to another? If only one or two gaps are responsible for the finding of insufficient evidence, it makes sense to tackle them first and then work on other gaps later to strengthen the recommendation and fill in additional details.

Equity

Existing health disparities are difficult to address in clinical prevention (AHRQ, 2018). These inequities arise from a number of complicated sociodemographic factors outside the scope of clinical practice, including inequitable distribution of resources, due to systems such as classism and racism that affect the social determinants of health. As a result, certain populations of individuals—particularly members of marginalized communities, such as racial and ethnic minorities—are less likely to receive high-quality services from the nation's health care system. It is vital that any additional medical research or development not add to this disadvantage and, if possible, that it work to make the health care system more equitable. Thus, researchers might give priority to those evidence gaps that, if addressed, could advance health equity. For example, in some cases, there has been uncertainty as to whether a preventive intervention is more or less effective for a particular population or racial group, because existing research has not included said population; as a matter of equity, research that addresses that uncertainty can be prioritized.

Relative Importance

Relative importance reflects the potential benefit the service could provide relative to other threats to health the patient population experiences. For example, screening a specific age group for a condition may continue to receive I statements despite updates because that age group has a high prevalence rate of other conditions or diseases. There are often competing risks to health in patient populations, and some may be determined as more important than others to the USPSTF, researchers, and funders.

Time Urgency

Some evidence gaps may be more urgent to address than others, particularly if they are foundational issues that affect the analytic framework evidence gaps. The effects of the interventions recommended by the USPSTF often play out over many years or even decades, and in these cases it may not make a major difference whether an evidence gap is addressed next year or 5 years from now. But depending on the burden of disease, some evidence gaps may be more pressing and thus more highly prioritized.

Adoptability

Some preventive services can be adopted more quickly and more widely than others, perhaps because of the nature of the intervention or of the population in which the intervention will take place.

Value, Including Economic Considerations

Stakeholders will also consider the value of the research that may fill an evidence gap. This question may be challenging because the value of the research depends in part on the value of the preventive service itself, and different approaches to estimating this value are possible. How does one value, for instance, research about a preventive service that is primarily intended to improve quality of life, compared with research about a preventive service that is primarily intended to increase life expectancy? There are various approaches to doing such valuations, and they can serve as the basis of estimating the cost-effectiveness of research aimed at closing different evidence gaps. When possible, priority should be given to the research that is most cost-effective.

Feasibility

Research studies that require unusually large study populations or expensive, time-consuming treatments of state-of-the-art measurements will be more difficult to carry out than those that require smaller populations, less expensive and less-labor-intensive treatments, and standard measurement techniques. The more feasible a study is, the faster and easier it will be to complete and the more likely it will be to be completed successfully. When prioritizing studies to address evidence gaps, priority should be given to those that are more feasible.

These prioritization considerations are not meant to be comprehensive. Instead they are intended to, first, bring attention to the importance of prioritizing research aimed at the various research gaps identified with the taxonomy and, second, to serve as a starting point for better lists that are more closely aligned with the goals of whatever organizations are doing the prioritization. Furthermore, as noted earlier, prioritization inevitably involves value judgments, so while the committee has come up with the foregoing list of considerations it finds to be most important, others will inevitably have their own opinions concerning what should be on the list. Of course, not every factor will have the same weight in determining a prioritization, and the weights used will vary from user to user and even sometimes from case to case. Some may value equity above all other considerations, for instance, while others may believe cost-effectiveness or population impact to be most important. The key here is to recognize that priorities must be set, to decide in a transparent way how priorities will be set, and then use that prioritization as a guide to which evidence gaps will be addressed first, second, and so forth.

Study Specification

The final step in developing a research agenda, after developing a taxonomy of evidence gaps and prioritizing those gaps is to decide on the details of the studies that will be required to fill in those gaps. This is not a novel process; indeed, it is one familiar to many investigators and funders. The approach to study specification is based on the PICOTS framework: population, intervention, comparison, outcome, timeframe, and setting

(FDA, n.d.). The committee added three more considerations important in specifying research aimed at filling in evidence gaps: Aggregability, design considerations, and potential funders and funding mechanisms (see Figure 4-10 for the corresponding workflow section). For many of the studies, effectiveness x risk and effectiveness x patient factors interactions will be important to assess. In designing such studies, suspected interactions (e.g., effectiveness differences) should be hypothesized a priori, and that purposive sampling may be necessary. Alternatively, sometimes the evidence gap will be within a subgroup, and that should perhaps be considered the entire study.

Each of those considerations is described briefly below.

Population

The proposed study design should explicitly define the population that will be the subject of the study. In determining the population, researchers should consider its relationship to the general affected population as well as how various individual factors may affect outcomes and lead to outcome differences across different individuals, particularly in the context of addressing health disparities and promoting health equity. The researchers should also explicitly define the selection criteria they will use and take into account any biases that may arise because of how the patients are selected or because of differences in patient attrition (FDA, n.d.).

Intervention

The investigators should define all of the components of the intervention and should make note of any factors that could influence the effectiveness or safety of the study, including such things as other treatments that took place before, during, or after the study and any specialized training of the provider of the intervention (FDA, n.d.).

Comparison Group

Concerning the comparison group, researchers should specify whether they are using a placebo or an active control for comparison. In the case of an active comparator it is best to use a comparator similar to what is currently being used in treatment of the disease or condition and to avoid any comparator that performs poorly in specific subpopulations (FDA, n.d.). It should also be ensured that the comparison group is as close as possible to receiving "usual care."

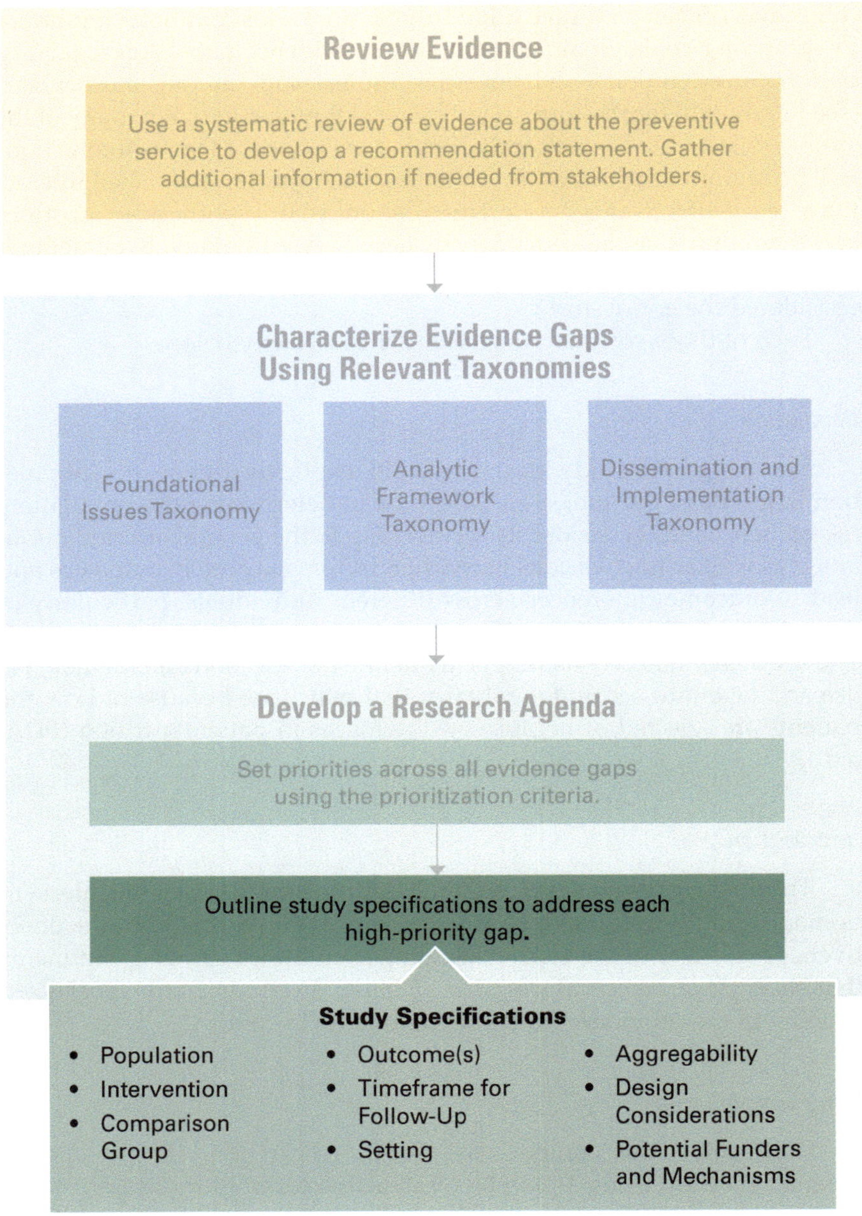

FIGURE 4-10 The workflow with study specifications facet.

Outcomes

In determining which safety and effectiveness outcomes to use, researchers should give preference to those that matter most to patients and that best predict successful results over the long term. Standard outcome measures should be recommended and used wherever possible. These measures may be defined based on measures used in prior studies, or may be selected based on accuracy or comprehensiveness in evaluating the important outcomes. Thoughtful selection of outcome measures will enhance the likelihood that each study can be compared or aggregated with past and future studies. Any surrogate outcomes should be clinically relevant. Researchers should determine ahead of time what outcome measures and analyses will be used, and the findings should be reported in terms of those predetermined measures and analyses, with any post hoc analyses clearly noted (FDA, n.d.).

Timeframe for Follow-Up

Researchers should determine the duration of treatment ahead of time as well as the timing of any follow-up. Ideally, both short-term and long-term outcomes will be included in the study (FDA, n.d.).

Setting

Possible settings include the offices of primary care or specialty providers, hospital inpatient clinics, and long-term care facilities, including nursing homes. The researchers should specify in which setting(s) the intervention will take place and explain why the study's setting is relevant to real-world use (FDA, n.d.).

Aggregability

Aggregability refers to how well a new study will combine with previous studies to get closer to a definitive answer to a question about preventive services. In some cases of insufficient evidence, the results of a new study can be combined with those of previous studies, resulting in aggregate data that are sufficient for the USPSTF or other bodies to issue a recommendation for a service. Aggregability should be considered when designing a study to address an evidence gap, and such considerations should be explicitly set forth in descriptions of the proposed study. However, aggregation should be done with care if the research findings are not considered robust.

Design Considerations

Design considerations for addressing research needs may involve selecting a randomized controlled trial, observational study design, or an appropriate novel research method (see Appendix B for more on novel research methods). Other factors for consideration may include anticipated internal and external validity and extrinsic factors like time urgency or logistical barriers. Other considerations may include high per-patient costs; sample size and power; and the possibility of heterogeneous effects on different subpopulations within the study.

Potential Funders and Mechanisms

Finally, the description of a study should discuss where funding may come from, including potential funders and funding mechanisms. By combining these prioritization and specification steps, researchers can develop a systematic approach to addressing relevant evidence gaps in the evidence base for preventive interventions. The goal, of course, is to address those gaps with well-designed, high-quality studies that have the greatest chance of closing the gaps and leading to new recommendations. AHRQ offers a useful guidance on what such studies should look like. Specifically, in a guidance on using the PICOTS framework to strengthen evidence gathered in clinical trials, AHRQ concluded that "trials that provide high strength of evidence" do the following:

- Study patients who are likely to be offered the intervention in everyday practice
- Examine clinical strategies and complexities that are more likely to be replicated in practice
- Measure the most relevant set of benefits and harms
- Have low risk of bias
- Have adequate power to address subgroups
- Directly compare interventions
- Include all important intended and unintended effects including adherence and tolerability (FDA, n.d.)

EXAMPLES OF APPLYING THE TAXONOMY TO I STATEMENTS

To illustrate how the taxonomy can be applied to make the USPSTF recommendations more systematic and consistent, the committee prepared several examples based on existing I statements. In reading over these examples, it is important to keep in mind that they are based on what was contained in the recommendation statements, supplemented by additional considerations suggested by committee members, and thus they are likely to be incomplete and perhaps contain some inaccuracies. In short, they are not meant to be taken literally as conclusions about the various evidence gaps but instead to serve as illustrations of how the USPSTF might proceed if it adopted the committee's taxonomy.

The committee did not map out research agendas to address the evidence gaps related to the I statement in large part because the results of the prioritization are likely to be different for each stakeholder who goes through the process. However, once evidence gaps have been identified, the committee believes that it should be relatively straightforward to prioritize the relevant evidence gaps and design experiments to fill in those gaps. In addition, actors outside the USPSTF will take those steps, and the main purpose of this report is to offer a process to identify evidence gaps for the USPSTF, so the examples offered in this section focus on the part of the framework that is directly applicable to the USPSTF's work.

Screening for Cognitive Impairment in Older Adults

The USPSTF has concluded, "Current evidence is insufficient to assess the balance of benefits and harms of screening for cognitive impairment in older adults" (USPSTF, 2020a). The following statements from the research needs and gaps section expand on what is needed to transform this I statement into a recommendation. (The letters following each are intended to make it easier to see how the statements from the USPSTF research needs and gaps section map onto statements in the committee's taxonomy.) See Box 4-2 for an example of the original evidence gaps described by the USPSTF in the cognitive impairment screening, and see Tables 4-1 through 4-3 for an example of those gaps mapped to the taxonomy (identified with the same letters as Box 4-2), along with additional suggestions of evidence gaps from this committee. A program screening for cognitive impairment has two components: the screening and the management of those patients (and caregivers) who screen positive. Management might include more formal testing and both pharmacologic and nonpharmacologic interventions. The evidence is that screening can detect cognitive impairment, but there may still be D&I issues related to screening. The recommendation is an I statement because of insufficient evidence on the benefits of treatment.

BOX 4-2
Evidence Gaps Identified by the U.S. Preventive Services Task Force for the Cognitive Impairment Screening Recommendation

- More research is needed on the effect of screening (***A***) and early detection (***B***) of cognitive impairment (mild cognitive impairment [MCI] and mild to moderate dementia) on important patient, caregiver, and societal outcomes, including decision making, advance planning, and caregiver outcomes.
- The body of evidence on screening and interventions for cognitive impairment would benefit from more consistent definitions (***C***) and reporting of outcomes (***D***) to allow comparisons across trials, especially from trials with longer-term follow-up.
- Studies are needed of the effects of caregiver or patient–caregiver dyad interventions on delay or prevention of institutionalization (***E***), and the effects of delay in institutionalization on caregivers (***F***).
- Research is needed on treatments that clearly affect the long-term clinical course of cognitive impairment (***G***). It is also important that studies on screening and interventions for cognitive impairment report harms and reasons for attrition of trial participants (***H***).

NOTE: Letters in italic added by the committee for identification purposes.
SOURCE: USPSTF, 2020a.

TABLE 4-1 Foundational Evidence Gaps in the Cognitive Impairment Recommendation

Condition Definition and Nomenclature	The body of evidence on screening and interventions for cognitive impairment would benefit from more consistent definitions ... to allow comparisons across trials, especially from trials with longer-term follow-up. (*C*)
Disease Processes	*Studies are needed to look for risk factors with better predictive validity for cognitive impairment. If these are found, further studies would be needed to see if identifying and treating these individuals can positively affect outcomes.*
Preventive Services	*Studies are needed on ways to improve the detection of those with early cognitive impairment who will respond to treatment.*
Development of Standards	The body of evidence on screening and interventions for cognitive impairment would benefit from more ... reporting of outcomes to allow comparisons across trials, especially from trials with longer-term follow-up. (*D*)
Psychometric Properties	

NOTE: Text in Roman font indicates recommendations issued by the USPSTF; text in italic indicates examples of evidence gaps suggested by this committee.

TABLE 4-2 Analytic Framework Gaps in the Cognitive Impairment Recommendation

Risk Assessment and Health Equity Considerations	
Early Detection	
Early Detection	
Intermediate Outcomes	
Effects of Treatment on Intermediate Outcomes	
Link Between Intermediate Outcomes and Morbidity or Mortality	
Effectiveness	
Effects of Screening on Reduced Morbidity or Mortality	Studies are needed of the effects of caregiver or patient–caregiver dyad interventions on delay or prevention of institutionalization (*E*), and the effects of delay in institutionalization on caregivers (*F*). More research is needed on the effect of screening (*A*) and early detection (*B*) of cognitive impairment (mild cognitive impairment and mild to moderate dementia) on important patient, caregiver, and societal outcomes, including decision making, advance planning, and caregiver outcomes.
Effects of Treatment on Morbidity or Mortality	Research is needed on treatments that clearly affect the long-term clinical course of cognitive impairment (*G*).
Harms	
Harms Associated with Screening	It is also important that studies on screening for cognitive impairment report harms and reasons for attrition of trial participants (*H*).
Harms Associated with Treatment	It is also important that studies on interventions for cognitive impairment report harms and reasons for attrition of trial participants (*H*).

TABLE 4-3 Dissemination and Implementation Evidence Gaps in the Cognitive Impairment Recommendation

Size	
Scope of Services, Including Cost	Identify potential problems in health system delivering full range of medications and behavioral interventions.
Scalability	
Sustainability	
Penetration of Program into the Intended Audience	Identify degree to which clinicians will add or have added screening to practice.
Implementation of the Scope of Services	Identify issues in implementing a complex, multi-modal intervention in clinical settings.
Participation in the Program	Identify barriers to patient participation in screening and likelihood of opting for or against treatment after a positive screen.
Effectiveness of the Program	

NOTE: For illustration in the D&I example, the committee chose to assume effectiveness of treatment.

Screening with Electrocardiograms for Atrial Fibrillation

In 2018, the USPSTF concluded, "The current evidence is insufficient to assess the balance of benefits and harms of screening for atrial fibrillation with electrocardiography" (ECG) (USPSTF, 2018a). A draft new recommendation statement for late 2021 is available for public comment, and includes the following evidence gaps (letters in parentheses were added by the committee) (USPSTF, 2021d):

- *Randomized trials enrolling asymptomatic persons that directly compare screening to usual care (**A**) and that assess both health outcomes (**B**) and harms (**C**) are needed to understand the balance of benefits and harms of screening for AF [atrial fibrillation]. It is important that screening trials enroll sufficient participants of both sexes and diverse racial/ethnic groups to enable assessment of whether the detection of AF (**D**) or the benefits (**E**) or harms (**F**) of screening vary in different population groups.*
- *More research is needed on how to best optimize the accuracy of screening tests or strategies for AF (**G**).*
- *Understanding the stroke risk associated with subclinical AF (**H**), how that risk varies with duration or burden of AF (**I**), and the potential*

benefit of anticoagulation therapy among persons with subclinical AF is an important research need (J).

The committee transformed this paragraph into a taxonomy of evidence gaps as indicated below. As before, the committee also included some additional suggested gaps (in italic), which they determined by examining each element of the taxonomy and asking whether there might be additional gaps overlooked by the USPSTF (see Tables 4-4 through 4-6).

One of the clear benefits of using this taxonomy is the way it provides a visual overview of the evidence gaps. Unlike the paragraphs on evidence gaps, the USPSTF's recommendation statement, which contains much of the same information, this structured taxonomy shows at a glance that there are a couple of foundational issues to address along with a large number of evidence gaps concerning the clinical application of the preventive services (i.e., the analytic framework). Thus, the taxonomy provides a "big picture" of the evidence gaps that can be drilled down into in order to get more details on the specifics of the gaps.

Finally, as noted in an earlier example, the structure of the taxonomy encourages a systematic approach to thinking about the evidence gaps that makes it possible to identify gaps that may have otherwise gone unremarked. In this case, the committee suggested a few additional evidence gaps identified using the taxonomy.

TABLE 4-4 Foundational Evidence Gaps in the Atrial Fibrillation Recommendation

Condition Definition and Nomenclature	
Disease Processes	
Preventive Services	The effectiveness of newer technologies capable of assessing pulse and heart rhythm as potential screening strategies should be evaluated (*E*).
Development of Standards	Understanding how to best optimize the accuracy of ECG interpretation (*D*).
Psychometric Properties	

TABLE 4-5 Analytic Framework Evidence Gaps in the Atrial Fibrillation Recommendation

Risk Assessment and Health Equity Considerations	
	Studies are needed as to whether subpopulations exist that are at greater risk or for whom the preventive service may be more effective.
Early Detection	
Early Detection	Direct comparison of screening and early detection with usual care and early detection is needed (*A*).
Intermediate Outcomes	
Effects of Treatment on Intermediate Outcomes	
Link Between Intermediate Outcomes and Morbidity or Mortality	Research is needed to understand the stroke risk associated with brief episodes of subclinical atrial fibrillation (*F*).
Effectiveness	
Effects of Screening on Reduced Morbidity or Mortality	Randomized trials enrolling asymptomatic persons that assess health outcomes and harms are needed to understand the balance of benefits and harms of screening for atrial fibrillation (*B*).
Effects of Treatment on Morbidity or Mortality	Understanding the potential benefits of anticoagulation therapy when risk is significant is an important research need (*G*). *The research should address the issue of whether benefits are similar across various populations.*
Harms	
Harms Associated with Screening	Randomized trials enrolling asymptomatic persons that assess harms are needed to understand the balance of benefits and harms of screening for atrial fibrillation (*C*).
Harms Associated with Treatment	

NOTE: Text in Roman font indicates recommendations issued by the USPSTF; text in italic indicates examples of evidence gaps suggested by this committee.

TABLE 4-6 Dissemination and Implementation Evidence Gaps in the Atrial Fibrillation Recommendation

Size	*Research is needed to assess frequency, duration, and degree of exertion required by patients who receive an ECG, compared with pulse palpitation and compared with usual care.*
Scope of Services, Including Cost	*Research is needed to assess the accessibility of screening with ECGs in adults.* *Research is also needed to assess the costs of ECG compared with other interventions.*
Scalability	*At which venues can ECG be deployed to screen for atrial fibrillation in order to reach a larger proportion of adults?*
Sustainability	*Identify the barriers to population-wide implementation*
Penetration of the Program into the Intended Audience	*Research is needed to assess if all individuals 65 and older have access to care for an ECG screening.* *Identify if there are equity issues caused by barriers to access to screening.*
Implementation of the Scope of Services	*Identify barriers to implementation in order to reach all adults in a given community.*
Participation in the Program	Identify reasons as to why not all adults participate in the screening.
Effectiveness of the Program	*Research is needed to assess if the rate of case finding significantly improved over other preventive services, such as pulse palpitation.*

REFERENCES

AHRQ (Agency for Healthcare Research and Quality). 2018. *Achieving health equity in preventive services: Systematic evidence review*. Effective Healthcare Program. https://effectivehealthcare.ahrq.gov/products/health-equity-preventive/protocol (accessed August 31, 2021).

Äikäs, A. H., N. P. Pronk, M. H. Hirvensalo, and P. Absetz. 2017. Does implementation follow design? A case study of a workplace health promotion program using the 4-S program design and the PIPE impact metric evaluation models. *Journal of Occupational and Environmental Medicine* 59(8):752–760.

Äikäs, A. H., P. Absetz, M. H. Hirvensalo, and N. P. Pronk. 2019. What can you achieve in 8 years? A case study on participation, effectiveness, and overall impact of a comprehensive workplace health promotion program. *Journal of Occupational and Environmental Medicine* 61(12):964–977.

Äikäs, A., P. Absetz, M. Hirvensalo, and N. Pronk. 2020. Eight-year health risks trend analysis of a comprehensive workplace health promotion program. *International Journal of Environmental Research and Public Health* 17(24):9426.

Asunta, P., H. Viholainen, T. Ahonen, and P. Rintala. 2019. Psychometric properties of observational tools for identifying motor difficulties: A systematic review. *BMC Pediatrics* 19(1):322.

Castrucci, B. C., and J. Auerbach. 2019. Meeting individual social needs falls short of addressing social determinants of health. *Health Affairs Blog*. https://www.healthaffairs.org/do/10.1377/hblog20190115.234942/full (accessed October 21, 2021).

Chou, R., A. Cantor, B. Zakher, J. P. Mitchell, and M. Pappas. 2014. *Prevention of dental caries in children younger than 5 years old: Systematic review to update the U.S. Preventive Services Task Force recommendation*. Evidence Synthesis, No. 104. Rockville, MD: Agency for Healthcare Research and Quality. https://www.ncbi.nlm.nih.gov/books/NBK202092/figure/ch2.f1 (accessed November 2, 2021).

Chou, R., C. Evans, A. Hoverman, C. Sun, T. Dana, C. Bougatsos, S. Grusing, and P.T. Korthuis. 2019. *Pre-Exposure prophylaxis for the prevention of HIV infection: A systematic review for the U.S. Preventive Services Task Force*. Evidence Synthesis, No. 178. Rockville, MD: Agency for Healthcare Research and Quality. https://doi.org/10.1001/jama.2019.2591 (accessed November 2, 2021).

CSDH (Committee on Social Determinants of Health). 2008. *Closing the gap in a generation: Health equity through action on the social determinants of health*. Geneva, Switzerland: World Health Organization. https://www.who.int/social_determinants/final_report/csdh_finalreport_2008.pdf (accessed October 21, 2021).

Davidson, K. W., A. R. Kemper, C. A. Doubeni, C. Tseng, M. A. Simon, M. Kubik, S. J. Curry, J. Mills, A. H. Krist, Q. Ngo-Metzger, and A. Borsky. 2020. Developing primary care-based recommendations for social determinants of health: Methods of the U.S. Preventive Services Task Force. *Annals of Internal Medicine* 173:461–467.

Davidson, K. W., A. H. Krist, C. Tseng, M. Simon, C. A. Doubeni, A. R. Kemper, M. Kubik, Q. Ngo-Metzger, J. Mills, and A. Borsky. 2021. Incorporation of social risk in US Preventive Services Task Force recommendations and identification of key challenges for primary care. *JAMA* 326(14):1410–1415.

Doubeni, C. A., M. Simon, and A. H. Krist. 2021. Addressing systemic racism through clinical preventive service recommendations from the US Preventive Services Task Force. *JAMA* 325(7):627–628.

FDA (U.S. Food and Drug Administration). n.d. *Using the PICOTS framework to strengthen evidence gathered in clinical trials—guidance from the AHRQ's Evidence-Based Practice Centers program*. https://www.fda.gov/media/109448/download (accessed July 14, 2021).

Harris, R. P., M. Helfand, S. H. Woolf, K. N. Lohr, C. D. Mulrow, S. M. Teutsch, and D. Atkins. 2001. Current methods of US preventive services task force: A review of process. *American Journal of Preventive Medicine* 20(3):21–35.

Hedden, H. 2016. *The accidental taxonomist*. 2nd ed. Medford, NJ: Information Today.

Klabunde, C. N., E. M. Ellis, J. Villani, E. Neilson, K. Schwartz, E. A. Vogt, and Q. Ngo-Metzger. 2021. Characteristics of scientific evidence informing changed U.S. Preventive Services Task Force insufficient evidence statements. *American Journal of Preventive Medicine*. https://www.sciencedirect.com/science/article/abs/pii/S0749379721004578 (accessed November 29, 2021).

Lappalainen, T., and D. G. MacArthur. 2021. From variant to function in human disease genetics. *Science* 373(6562):1464–1468. https://www.science.org/doi/full/10.1126/science.abi8207 (accessed November 2, 2021).

Mabry-Hernandez, I. R., S. J. Curry, W. R. Phillips, F. A. García, K. W. Davidson, J. W. Epling, Q. Ngo-Metzger, A. S. Bierman. 2018. U.S. Preventive Services Task Force priorities for prevention research. *American Journal of Preventive Medicine* 54(1 Suppl 1):S95–S103.

MacDonald, A. J., H. McEwan, M. McCabe, and A. Macdonald. 2011. Age at death of patients with colorectal cancer and the effect of lead-time bias on survival in elective vs emergency surgery. *Colorectal Disease* 13(5):519–525.

Pronk, N. P. 2003. Designing and evaluating health promotion programs: Simple rules for a complex issue. *Disease Management and Health Outcomes* 11(3):149–157.

USPSTF (U.S. Preventive Services Task Force). 2013. *Glaucoma: Screening*. https://www.uspreventiveservicestaskforce.org/uspstf/recommendation/glaucoma-screening (accessed October 21, 2021).

USPSTF. 2016a. *Breast cancer: Screening.* https://www.uspreventiveservicestaskforce.org/uspstf/recommendation/breast-cancer-screening (accessed August 17, 2021).

USPSTF. 2016b. *Depression in adults: Screening.* https://www.uspreventiveservicestaskforce.org/uspstf/recommendation/depression-in-adults-screening (accessed October 26, 2021).

USPSTF. 2017. *Celiac disease: Screening.* https://www.uspreventiveservicestaskforce.org/uspstf/recommendation/celiac-disease-screening (accessed July 14, 2021).

USPSTF. 2018a. *Atrial fibrillation: Screening with electrocardiography.* https://www.uspreventiveservicestaskforce.org/uspstf/draft-recommendation/screening-atrial-fibrillation (accessed August 17, 2021).

USPSTF. 2018b. *Child maltreatment: Interventions.* https://www.uspreventiveservicestaskforce.org/uspstf/recommendation/child-maltreatment-primary-care-interventions (accessed November 2, 2021).

USPSTF. 2018c. *Grade definitions.* https://www.uspreventiveservicestaskforce.org/uspstf/about-uspstf/methods-and-processes/grade-definitions (accessed November 2, 2021).

USPSTF. 2019. *Prevention of human immunodeficiency virus (HIV) infection: Preexposure prophylaxis.* https://www.uspreventiveservicestaskforce.org/uspstf/recommendation/prevention-of-human-immunodeficiency-virus-hiv-infection-pre-exposure-prophylaxis#bootstrap-panel--6 (accessed October 19, 2021).

USPSTF. 2020a. Screening for cognitive impairment in older adults. *JAMA* 323(8):757–763.

USPSTF. 2020b. *Unhealthy drug use: Screening.* https://www.uspreventiveservicestaskforce.org/uspstf/recommendation/drug-use-illicit-screening (accessed August 17, 2021).

USPSTF. 2021a. *Hypertension in adults: Screening.* https://www.uspreventiveservicestaskforce.org/uspstf/recommendation/hypertension-in-adults-screening (accessed October 26, 2021).

USPSTF. 2021b. *Chlamydia and gonorrhea: Screening.* https://www.uspreventiveservicestaskforce.org/uspstf/recommendation/chlamydia-and-gonorrhea-screening (accessed November 2, 2021).

USPSTF. 2021c. *Procedure manual section 3: Topic workplan development.* https://www.uspreventiveservicestaskforce.org/uspstf/about-uspstf/methods-and-processes/procedure-manual/procedure-manual-section-3-topic-work-plan-development (accessed October 25, 2021).

USPSTF. 2021d. *Screening for atrial fibrillation: Draft recommendation statement.* https://www.uspreventiveservicestaskforce.org/uspstf/draft-update-summary/screening-atrial-fibrillation (accessed November 2, 2021).

USPSTF. 2021e. *Tobacco smoking cessation in adults, including pregnant persons: Interventions.* https://www.uspreventiveservicestaskforce.org/uspstf/recommendation/tobacco-use-in-adults-and-pregnant-women-counseling-and-interventions (accessed August 17, 2021).

Wolff, T. A., A. H. Krist, M. LeFevre, D. E. Jonas, R. P. Harris, A. Siu, D. K. Owens, M. W. Gillman, M. H. Ebell, J. Herzstein, R. Chou, E. Whitlock, and K. Bibbins-Domingo. 2018. Update on the methods of the US Preventive Services Task Force: Linking intermediate outcomes and health outcomes in prevention. *American Journal of Preventive Medicine* 54(1S1):S4–S10. https://doi.org/10.1016/j.amepre.2017.08.032 (accessed November 2, 2021).

5

Recommendations

The committee makes eight recommendations in three categories: using the taxonomy developed in Chapter 4, fostering clinical prevention research, and advancing the work of the U.S. Preventive Services Task Force (USPSTF). The rationale for each recommendation follows the recommendation text itself. The chapter and report end with the committee's vision.

USING THE TAXONOMY

Chapter 4 describes a taxonomy for use in systematically describing evidence gaps in three facets: foundational research, the analytic framework used by the USPSTF, and dissemination and implementation (D&I). The committee also outlines two additional facets to guide the process for developing a research agenda: prioritizing evidence gaps and outlining key research studies. Embedded throughout this process is the opportunity to elevate evidence gaps pertaining to recommendations that promote health equity. The committee envisions identifying and prioritizing evidence gaps as the responsibility of the USPSTF with assistance from staff from the Agency for Healthcare Research and Quality (AHRQ) and the National Institutes of Health's (NIH's) Office of Disease Prevention (ODP) and other stakeholders, including but not limited to the USPSTF partner organizations. The committee developed Recommendations 1 and 2 with the work of the USPSTF in mind but hopes that other prevention guideline developers find this useful and adopt it. The committee understands that successfully implementing these recommendations will take time, staff, training, and other resources, and encourages AHRQ and NIH to begin planning their implementation as soon as possible. Recommendation 3 is directed at AHRQ and NIH to maintain and update the taxonomy.

Characterizing Evidence Gaps

Recommendation 1: For each of its recommendation statements, the U.S. Preventive Services Task Force should use the Clinical Prevention Research Taxonomy to identify and describe evidence gaps.

The USPSTF will likely and understandably be most inclined to focus their efforts on the analytic framework evidence gaps, as it is already a part of their process. These evidence gaps emerge from the evidence review provided by an Evidence-based Practice Center (EPC) and the USPSTF deliberations (AHRQ, 2018). As noted in Chapters 2 and 4, each USPSTF recommendation statement includes a section titled "Research Needs and Gaps," and the text of these sections has grown more specific in recent years. Framing the research needs around the terms within the taxonomy will impart consistency in the USPSTF efforts to describe research needs. The committee notes that while it is important for the USPSTF to articulate what evidence gaps exist, at least one I statement mentioned research that is not needed (USPSTF, 2018a). That information is likely very helpful to researchers and to funders. Although this recommendation does not refer to EPCs, it is nonetheless envisioned that AHRQ will direct EPCs to conduct reviews using terminology consistent with the taxonomy.

The USPSTF can also use the taxonomy to identify foundational research gaps. As described in Chapters 2 and 4, the basis for some I statements rests on the inability of the EPC and the USPSTF to use the analytic framework due to a lack of common understanding among researchers and clinicians regarding definitions of the condition, accepted and standardized diagnoses and treatments, or simple mechanistic information about how and when a condition leads to adverse health outcomes. As an example, the research need section in the USPSTF statement about screening for child maltreatment states, "Further research to determine effective methods for clinicians to identify children at increased risk should be a priority" (USPSTF, 2018b). Other recommendations lack evidence on groups disproportionately affected by the condition or on the specifics of the preventive service.

Dissemination and Implementation Gaps

AHRQ has a robust implementation portfolio. While the USPSTF has not had D&I of recommendations as its remit, it has recognized the importance of D&I research. The first annual report to Congress issued in 2011 identified "Gaps in Implementation Research" as follows (USPSTF, 2011, p. 13):

1. How do primary care professionals incorporate new evidence to change their practice?
2. What are the most effective strategies to assist primary care professionals in the translation of evidence-based clinical preventive services into practice?
3. How can primary care professionals share evidence with their patients to empower patients and families to make health care decisions about prevention?
4. How can health information technology, including electronic health records and personal health records, be utilized to increase the number of Americans receiving recommended clinical preventive services?
5. How can the USPSTF continue to improve its work to better meet the needs of primary care professionals and their patients?

More recently, AHRQ staff and the USPSTF members wrote,

> Although the use of implementation research is not within the scope of the USPSTF's deliberations, it notes that there are critical questions about how to best implement recommended clinical preventive services in primary care practices. Additional implementation and translational research will increase the value of the USPSTF's work and would be helpful in its deliberations. (Mabry-Hernandez et al., 2018)

Because the committee was not tasked with recommending how the USPSTF determines its recommendations, it does not intend that dissemination and implementation considerations would influence the letter grade recommendations issued by the USPSTF. However, it is clear from the request from AHRQ and ODP to the National Academies of Sciences, Engineering, and Medicine and from the discussions with the committee in open sessions, that the committee was encouraged to address clinical prevention research needs writ large (NASEM, 2020). Ignoring dissemination and implementation issues could mean that important preventive services are not deployed.

There is not currently a body tasked with ensuring that the USPSTF recommendations are adopted in practice, although the requirement in the Patient Protection and Affordable Care Act that A and B recommendations be covered at no cost to patients is an important tool (KFF, 2015). The Guide to Community Preventive Services, discussed in Chapter 2, deals with some of the same topics as the USPSTF, focusing on population-based interventions, but their remit is much broader than the clinical preventive services the USPSTF addresses. Additionally, Murad et al. (2021) recently proposed the consideration of contextual and implementation evidence as part of a five-prong approach to supplementing systematic review findings when evidence is insufficient for decision making. The authors explain, "Evidence on other factors that may affect the decision may be helpful to decision makers, such as patient values, equity, resources, acceptability, and feasibility" (Murad et al., 2021). For example, the USPSTF updated its lung cancer screening recommendation to lower pack years and age for initiating screening (USPSTF, 2021c). This revised recommendation may promote health equity by identifying Black men who are at greater risk for lung cancer relative to white men (Doubeni et al., 2021). Dissemination and implementation approaches could also address known inequities in screening access, screening quality, time to treatment, and treatment quality (Doubeni et al., 2021).

There are several ways the work related to the D&I of the USPSTF recommendations could be accomplished. The committee hopes that eventually the USPSTF will assume responsibility for the D&I work, agreeing with the USPSTF members and AHRQ staff who acknowledge that it will be helpful in their work (Mabry-Hernandez et al., 2018). However, the committee understands that the USPSTF carries a large workload and that this requires time and resources to be fully implemented. In the short term, partner organizations and staff at AHRQ and ODP could provide pivotal support and input. Other important partners for working on D&I include AHRQ staff who do not already provide scientific and technical support to USPSTF; the Centers for Disease Control and Prevention (CDC), particularly the Community Guide and the Prevention Research Center networks; NIH staff tasked with implementation research; the Patient-Centered Outcomes Research Institutes; and representatives of professional provider organizations, such as the American Academy of Family Physicians or the American Academy of Pediatrics.

As with foundational and analytic framework evidence gaps, addressing D&I will involve information gathering, identification of evidence gaps, and a research agenda addressing priority gaps. For the evidence review, AHRQ could broaden the request to the EPC doing the evidence review for the recommendation statement or engage a different group. The evidence review and identification of evidence gaps could range from an extremely thorough process and report, similar to the evidence reviews that underpin the current USPSTF recommendations, to a more top-level summary of key issues derived from workshops with stakeholders, for example. EPCs could comment on the D&I challenges, particularly those that affect health equity, with input from their review author teams and stakeholders. Regardless of who performs the evidence review and identifies the D&I evidence gaps, the committee has provided a taxonomy for use. The committee envisions that the USPSTF will be sufficiently supported and resourced to be involved in and informed by this activity. Nevertheless, the committee acknowledges that this work will take time, staff, and other resources.

For some recommendation topics, there will be scant information on dissemination and implementation. For others, such as recommendations that address an expanded age range for an already recommended intervention (as with lung cancer screening), or an intervention already widely used in practice despite the recommendation grade, there could be a great deal of existing information and expertise available from the provider community. D&I issues might also be similar for certain types of interventions. For example, the implementation issues for administering brief questionnaires are likely to be similar, regardless of the specific topic. In addition, implementation issues around preventive services requiring costly equipment will likely have features in common, and referring patients based on screening results to community resources will likely have common or overlapping D&I issues as well. Those interested in describing gaps related to dissemination and implementation work might start with an effort to outline common themes or challenges in implementation to facilitate the work on specific I statements.

Emerging technological advances for discrete steps in the systematic review process, such as artificial intelligence, can revolutionize the efficiency of systematic review production and updating (Lau, 2019). For example, living systematic reviews, which incorporate findings from research studies as they become available, are also emerging as a strategy (Elliott et al., 2017; McDonagh et al., 2021). As another example, a machine learning-based routine has been developed to distinguish between randomized controlled trials (RCTs), quasi-randomized trials, and non-randomized studies (Marshall et al., 2018). Others can extract PICO (population, intervention, comparison, outcomes) information, study design and results, and risk of bias information (Jonnalagadda et al., 2015). These methods could potentially facilitate a less burdensome review of D&I evidence.

It is important to recognize the iterative nature of the assessment of the analytic framework evidence and the D&I evidence, even with I statements. Postponing a review of information on dissemination and implementation until a letter grade recommendation of A or B is made by the USPSTF presents potential problems. Should the D&I evidence review suggest that the barriers to adoption and spread of the intervention are great, the USPSTF and others might not prioritize filling analytic framework gaps. Alternatively, D&I research might suggest insufficient evidence for a complex intervention, yet sufficient evidence for a simpler intervention. The USPSTF and others may use this information when evaluating the intervention (a less effective intervention that can be implemented easily may be preferred over a more effective intervention that cannot be implemented). Additionally, appropriately targeted research on dissemination and implementation, if not funded or conducted until after an intervention receives a letter grade of A or B, will lag, and the needs of practitioners and patients will suffer.

Given the demands on the USPSTF members and on the EPCs, a full articulation by the USPSTF of D&I evidence gaps might not be possible, particularly at the time of the publication of the recommendation or I statement. When these evidence gaps are articulated, regardless by whom, the USPSTF recommendation statement page could link to the information, even if it is not authored by the USPSTF.

The committee's task was primarily focused on the USPSTF; however, the committee hopes that other guideline developers working in prevention will consider using the taxonomy provided. Consistency in framing research questions about a specific intervention could lead to synergies in research agendas and research funding and thereby advance health equity. AHRQ and ODP can post the taxonomy prominently on their websites so that others can use it.

Developing a Research Agenda

> **Recommendation 2: For each recommendation and I statement, the U.S. Preventive Services Task Force (USPSTF) should indicate high-priority evidence gaps. Staff from the Office of Disease Prevention (ODP) in the National Institutes of Health and from the Agency for Healthcare Research and Quality (AHRQ) should broadly outline research that could address those priority gaps and be available to help funders, whether NIH or others, develop a research agenda to address them. The USPSTF and staff from ODP and AHRQ should consult partner organizations and stakeholders as needed.**

The committee was asked to provide a taxonomy of evidence gaps and has done so; however, as described in Chapters 1 and 4, the committee was also urged to facilitate prioritizing the evidence gaps. In order to make those priorities evident and actionable by funders and researchers, the committee outlines two steps in the development of a research agenda: identifying priority gaps related to a specific recommendation or

I statement and broadly outlining research to address priority evidence gaps.

Prioritization

The committee acknowledges that formal prioritization exercises can be difficult and burdensome and might require additional resources to support this activity. Nevertheless, the committee believes that any description of evidence gaps in foundational issues or the analytic framework should include a discussion of the priorities. Two I statements in the last 5 years reference a research need as a "priority," so this is not completely anathema to the USPSTF (2017, 2018b). The USPSTF members are best suited to prioritize evidence gaps, especially regarding foundational research and analytic framework gaps.

As above regarding the USPSTF role in reviewing D&I evidence, the committee suggests that, given the demands on the USPSTF members, identifying priority gaps and outlining research to fill those gaps could be done by AHRQ staff and ODP and other NIH staff in *consultation with* the USPSTF members and stakeholders. If there are concerns about this process holding up issuance of a USPSTF recommendation statement, this could be published separately and subsequent to publication of the recommendation statement itself.

A structured method for setting priorities would be an important enhancement of the committee's approach but is beyond the remit and expertise of the committee. However, AHRQ and NIH could embark on this project. Examples of such structured approaches to prioritization include rating, ranking, voting, multi-criteria decision analysis, analytic hierarchy process; and value of information. Iterative dialogue among stakeholders will be important in this process, regardless of the approach chosen. Until such methods are tested and deployed, those setting USPSTF-related research priorities can use the prioritization criteria terms in the committee's taxonomy qualitatively or perhaps selectively.

The USPSTF might initially focus on "centrality," rather than prioritizing using all of the criteria proposed. The USPSTF has recently committed to "advancing its methods to better identify when systemic racism contributes to health inequities and to include evidence-based strategies that will reverse the negative effects of systemic racism on preventable disease" (Doubeni et al., 2021, p. 628). As such, the committee anticipates that the USPSTF members might also consider health equity as a prioritization criterion. The committee further urges that whoever takes on the responsibility for prioritizing dissemination and implementation evidence gaps think broadly about the stakeholders it involves, to include practitioners who disproportionately care for patients with the condition, and to include patients themselves.

It should be emphasized that prioritized evidence gaps may not and should not only emerge from I statements. The USPSTF includes research needs for all populations singled out in recommendation statements, not just I statements. Research needs for a specific subgroup might be prioritized as more important to address than the research needs that apply to a different subgroup within the same recommendation statement. For example, the USPSTF recommends chlamydia and gonorrhea screening for women with a B grade, while there is an I statement for screening for men (USPSTF, 2021a). Current evidence gaps note that the prevalence of disease is high among American Indian/Alaska Native, Black, Hispanic/Latino, and Native Hawaiian/Pacific Islander persons. When developing a research agenda for this recommendation statement, groups like AHRQ, NIH, and the USPSTF will need to consider how to prioritize research addressing racial and ethnic health disparities compared with the dearth of evidence regarding screening men in general for chlamydia or gonorrhea.

The committee has not addressed the important issue of prioritizing *across* recommendation statements. The prioritization facet would be useful for that as well. As the AHRQ, NIH, the USPSTF, and stakeholders gain experience prioritizing *within* a recommendation statement, they could indicate priorities across topics. The annual reports to Congress would be a natural place for such efforts to emerge.

The prioritization taxonomy is useful for many purposes and might result in different priority rankings when applied by different stakeholders. The USPSTF should use it to signal to funders the evidence gaps it most needs addressed to improve its ability to offer recommendations for clinical practice. Funders might come to different priorities using the same criteria because of differences in focus or mission. For example, a funder who has prioritized advancing equity in their mission might choose to invest in those evidence gaps for which evidence is missing regarding disadvantaged populations. A funder specifically interested in advancing women's health might choose to invest in evidence gaps that focus on women as a subpopulation about whom more information is needed.

Outlining Research

One of the frustrations identified by stakeholders is that the USPSTF research needs have not usually been specific with regard to some key elements of study design, such as whether an RCT is required. As described in Chapter 4, the committee provides a taxonomy of study specifications, an elaboration of the standard PICOTS (population, intervention, comparison, outcome, timing, setting) framework, which should be considered by whomever completes the research agenda. The enhancements of the PICOTS framework include aggregability, design considerations, and potential funders and funding mechanisms. In particular, the committee urges ODP and AHRQ staff, when outlining research to address the prioritized gaps, to consider these three enhancements. Aggregability is important for building a robust dataset for the USPSTF to consider in the future. NIH staff in the Institutes and Centers (ICs) interested in supporting research addressing USPSTF gaps could also consider whether the newly funded studies can be pooled with existing evidence.

Detailed design considerations could be left up to those submitting research proposals, but if the USPSTF or others outlining the research agenda think an RCT is or is not necessary, they should so state. Since 2018, the USPSTF has specifically called for an RCT in four I statement research need sections (USPSTF, 2018c, 2019, 2021b,d). Another I statement calls out the need for research that would allow for better pooling of new data (USPSTF, 2020). The importance of and rationale for specifying potential funding mechanisms are addressed in Recommendation 6.

The committee urges that each item in the specification facet be considered, but that the research agenda not be overly prescriptive, so as not to limit researcher creativity or funders' expectations of research proposals. Appendix B includes a discussion of study designs that AHRQ and ODP staff, funders, and researchers can consider when outlining studies for a USPSTF-focused research agenda.

Institutionalizing the Use of the Taxonomy

Recommendation 3: The National Institutes of Health and the Agency for Healthcare Research and Quality should make the taxonomy accessible on their websites and integrate the taxonomy terms and phrases in their relevant publications, including but not limited to the U.S. Preventive Services Task Force recommendation statements, funding announcements, and grant and contract awards.

The goal is to make the taxonomy and workflow accessible to the clinical prevention community and the public at large. Consistent use of these metadata will provide a common language to stakeholders and encourage wider adoption of the taxonomy. Applying the taxonomy terms in publications linking USPSTF recommendations or I statements with funding opportunity announcements will be crucial for making evident the impact of the research agenda laid out by the USPSTF.

In order to ensure relevance and usability, the taxonomy and workflow will need to be maintained, updated, and evaluated. Maintenance of the taxonomy includes logistics such as documentation, formatting, and sharing with other stakeholders. Updating and evaluating the taxonomy and workflow require subject-matter expertise to assess and modify terms to reflect the needs and experiences of the users. It is not unusual for taxonomies to undergo regular updates. AHRQ and ODP staff are well placed to advise on this. Encouraging wide use of the taxonomy means that the taxonomy must be shared; thus, AHRQ and ODP are encouraged to post the taxonomy on their websites.

FOSTERING CLINICAL PREVENTION RESEARCH

The committee was asked to propose ways for prevention research funders and guideline developers to enhance their partnership to accelerate research to close important gaps in prevention. A robust and relevant research agenda requires funding, funding requests that are clear and clearly linked to USPSTF research needs, and appropriate mechanisms for and oversight of funded research. As such, the committee provides recommendations regarding the funding and commissioning of clinical prevention research.

Recommendation 4: Funders, in particular the National Institutes of Health and the Patient-Centered Outcomes Research Institute, should set aside funding to address high-priority evidence gaps identified by the U.S. Preventive Services Task Force.

In order to act in a timely manner on a research agenda for clinical prevention developed by the USPSTF, AHRQ staff and ODP and other NIH staff, EPCs, and other stakeholders, dedicated funding will be needed. NIH and stakeholders can work with Congress and the U.S. Department of Health and Human Services leadership to identify appropriate funding levels and secure sufficient funding for this area of need. This funding might be identified and managed at the IC level or at the level of the Office of the Director, or both. Many research questions may require trans-institute collaboration, and these should be actively encouraged. Managing large, directive research, such as called for in Recommendation 4, requires program staff with specialized expertise and the remit to focus on this important task.

The committee acknowledges that calls for increased funding for prevention research have been made by others in the past and not always successfully. However, as described in Chapter 3, NIH's budget, while never large enough to satisfy all stakeholders, is approximately $41.7 billion and in 2016 only 20 percent of that was, at best, spent on prevention research, broadly defined (Murray, 2017; NIH, 2020). The amount devoted to clinical prevention research of direct relevance to the USPSTF is undoubtedly much less.

Recommendation 5: The National Institutes of Health staff developing funding announcements for research related to high-priority evidence gaps should consult with the Office of Disease Prevention and the Agency for Healthcare Research and Quality to ensure appropriateness of support mechanisms and fidelity to the research specifications and should include a link to the research needs document on the U.S. Preventive Services Task Force website.

Program announcements; notices of special interest; requests for applications or proposals; and research opportunity announcements related to high-priority research needs of importance to the USPSTF should be as explicit as possible to ensure usefulness to the USPSTF and other guideline developers. AHRQ and ODP staff could serve as an important resource in the crafting of the requests and notices. Reviewers of applications and proposals could be encouraged to study the research needs specification from the USPSTF. Study sections dedicated to these applications could ensure that study section members are oriented to the needs of the USPSTF. As discussed in Chapter 2, although much of the evidence used to establish a letter grade recommendation uses RCT designs, not all important studies do. Given the expense of RCTs, when the research agenda suggests other designs, the funding announcements should so note.

Recommendation 6: The National Institutes of Health and other funders addressing high-priority clinical prevention evidence gaps identified by the U.S. Preventive Services Task Force should use funding mechanisms and processes that can assure that research is conducted expediently, efficiently, and with fidelity to the specified research needs, rather than waiting for such research needs to be addressed predominantly through investigator-initiated grant mechanisms.

The committee encourages NIH and other funders to explore developing creative new programs that can be brought to bear on closing evidence gaps in clinical prevention. For example, NIH's Clinical and Translational Science Awards (CTSA) program aims to improve the efficiency, quality, and impact of turning research observations into interventions. Their history of supporting multi-disciplinary teams working toward very specific goals is the sort of program that could be used to help close the USPSTF priority evidence gaps. NIH supports a federally funded research and development center. This very directed and focused mechanism might be used to build out contracted clinical prevention research. Expanding and establishing trans-NIH prevention interests into networks for clinical prevention research could also contribute to closing high-priority evidence gaps identified by the USPSTF by establishing an infrastructure to conduct prevention research. Activities would include dataset curation, survey researchers, modelers, and clinical trial infrastructure that would be poised to respond to calls to fill evidence gaps. Such a network would complement CDC's Prevention Research Centers, discussed in Chapter 3. As a complement to its work described in Chapter 3 regarding I statement surveys, ODP could serve as the consultant to and coordinator of these directed research efforts.

As discussed in Chapter 3, a recent analysis of research that was used to upgrade a USPSTF recommendation from an I Statement to an A or B recommendation indicates that contract mechanisms were key to resolving three I statements (Klabunde et al., 2021). A contract, or other directive funding mechanism (e.g., Other Transaction Authority Cooperative Agreements), can increase the likelihood that studies are of sufficient design; to allow for aggregating studies; to demonstrate an effect, if the intervention indeed is effective; and to meet the methodologic rigor for high-quality studies identified in the USPSTF evidence syntheses. Regular consultation with the awardees could ensure that the research is being conducted in a timely manner with fidelity to the research needs specification.

As discussed in Chapter 3, NIH has programs that are specifically designed to stimulate technological innovation. Programs such as Small Business Innovation Research (SBIR) or Small Business Technology Transfer (SBTT) could encourage private enterprise to engage in appropriate clinical prevention research. ODP and AHRQ staff could undertake outreach activities to such firms when a high-priority research need involves the development of new technologies.

ADVANCING THE WORK OF THE U.S. PREVENTIVE SERVICES TASK FORCE

The committee understands the immensity of the workload of the USPSTF, the rigor with which the members adhere to the advice of methodologists, and the importance of consistency of approach across time. The committee's recommendations are based on a combination of evidence explained in Chapter 2 and familiarity with the work of the USPSTF and other guideline developers. As such, the committee makes recommendations intended to enhance and advance the work of the USPSTF and other guideline developers in order for them to provide as many definitive recommendations for practice as possible, and to ensure that the recommendations lead to improved health of the target population.

> **Recommendation 7: The Agency for Healthcare Research and Quality should fund research in how guideline developers assess evidence and issue clinical practice guidelines, including how the decision of "insufficient evidence" is made and how a committee decides which research gaps are the key.**

Most evidence-based clinical practice guidelines (CPGs) include a statement on the level of the evidence and a separate statement on the strength of the recommendation. The USPSTF combines these two attributes into a "Level of Certainty." Simply stating a Level of Certainty, or even separately stating a level of evidence and strength of the recommendation, obscures much of the decision making that occurs when translating the evidence into a recommendation. In other words, an evidence-based guideline may be explicit in terms of the methods for evaluating the level of evidence, but not explicit in how the guideline developer uses many factors to determine not only the strength of the recommendation but also the recommendation itself.

This is important because different groups looking at the same topic can issue different guidelines for practice. Sometimes this is because they look at different data (an accidentally incomplete literature review or a review that is purposefully limited by language, years of publication, study type, etc.). Regardless, if two guideline developers look at the same body of evidence, CPGs will still vary, as they are also informed by differences in the *dynamics* of the guideline developers, different biases among or between the guideline developers, and differences in considerations used to determine the guideline. These considerations might include

- the types of outcomes (e.g., primary outcomes of a trial versus primary and secondary, including side effects),
- the balance of benefits and harms,
- opportunities for shared decision making (including recognizing cultural differences), or
- the incorporation of elements of equity.

Different guideline developers arriving at different recommendations can lead to several problems. For one, there is the confusion for the clinicians and patients as to which guideline should be followed. That two guideline developers arrive at a different recommendation raises the questions, Which is right?, Is either right?, Might they both be right? In addition, CPGs with differing recommendations can lead to a questioning of the process and its validity: Should any guideline be followed? The confusion might also lead payers to wonder which, if any, guideline practice to reimburse.

In addition, there is the question of evidence threshold. How much evidence is needed for a topic to receive a letter grade and become a CPG? Again, this is subjective and will vary not only between CPG panels but on different guideline statements from one panel. This is because many factors (evidence, benefit–harm balance, group dynamics, bias, tradition, and much more) all interplay in this decision.

There are many potential solutions for these problems. One solution is for guideline developers to be even more explicit in their rationales. For example, Rosenfeld et al. (2013) proposed an explicit profile that should accompany each recommendation. The authors proposed that several factors play into the final "strength of recommendation" decision, including the quality of the evidence, the benefits, the risks/harms/costs, the benefit–harm assessment, value judgments, intentional vagueness, role of patient preferences, and others. This level of detail helps make the decision-making process of guideline developers more explicit, and could potentially clarify why two guideline developers might arrive at different conclusions regarding the same topic. These factors are not always clearly defined. For example, one of the factors identified by Rosenfield et al. (2013) is "Risks, harms, cost." A component of "Risk, harms, cost" might include how each of those are counted in the future. In addition to these factors that supplement the evidence base during guideline development, guideline developers might also consider advancing health equity, achieving successful dissemination and implementation, and improving public health.

This complexity leads to another potential solution. In addition to being more explicit in the thought process supporting a guideline, it is important to better understand *the process of group decision making* by guideline developers. Balancing the large number of factors and data relevant for a given CPG may be difficult for an individual, and this is made more difficult when each individual brings their own expertise, experiences, and conscious and unconscious biases to a group discussion. At times, more influential than the evidence reviewed might be *how the committee works*. This means there are many questions on what determines which data the committee chooses to look at, how it evaluates the data, how it balances the different elements of the evidence base, how the dynamics of the committee affect the final assessment. These questions are not evidence gaps, but they are important questions that, if addressed, can improve guideline fidelity and quality. Increasing the knowledge of the processes of group decision making may lead to methods for improving this task.

Recommendation 8: The Agency for Healthcare Research and Quality should work with relevant government agencies and key stakeholders to evaluate how effectively U.S. Preventive Services Task Force recommendations are implemented in real-world settings to identify and address gaps in achieving the intended benefits.

Simply making a recommendation may not have the intended impact on clinical care and population health, and in fact, may lead to widening health disparities—particularly if there are underlying differences in access and quality of screening and care. Evaluation of programs suggested by a recommendation can occur for both process and health outcomes. These evaluations ask if outcomes improve after the guideline is disseminated or implemented. For example, do colorectal cancer screenings increase after the guideline is published (process outcome); does colorectal cancer death decrease after the guideline is published (clinical outcome); or are some groups disproportionately benefiting after a recommendation while others lag behind (process and clinical outcome) (Davidson et al., 2021)?

Program evaluation has been defined as the systematic definition of the merit, worth, and significance of a program, project, or policy (Adams and Neville, 2020). The methods, models, and theories of evaluation science are diverse (Frye and Hemmer, 2012), but the abiding questions are those of determining (in the case of a preventive or other clinical intervention program that has been recommended) the program's benefits, its harms, who it benefits, and what it costs. Many questions are addressed and provisionally answered in the initial efficacy studies, but as these programs are promulgated, implemented, and disseminated over time, questions related to effectiveness should arise. A primary question is how a program's "real-world" outcomes compare to those of the initial trials. The outcomes may change because of training (practitioners in real-world settings may be trained and incentivized differently than those in a trial) and there may not be sufficient fiscal and skilled personnel resources available. This may lead to a program that is implemented differently than the program that was evaluated in the efficacy studies. In addition, underlying technologies and protocols may change, as may the target populations or the disease natural histories. All these factors may influence the effectiveness of the program's implementation.

Some important evaluation research is being conducted. For example, in a study of colorectal cancer in 21 European countries, divergent mortality rates are related to the extent of screening program implementation (Cardoso et al., 2021). Staff from CDC and NIH collaborate on studies using data from national surveys to analyze temporal trends in the use of cancer screening tests (Hall et al., 2018). In another example, in an evaluation of a meta-analysis and new RCTs, it was concluded that low-dose computed tomography for lung cancer screening does continue to improve survivorship in high-risk persons (Manuel et al., 2021), as reported in the original USPSTF guideline.

Still, despite the professed need for periodic evaluation programs of all important and commonly applied interventions, evaluation challenges remain. In the context of evaluating federal programs, Orr suggested three important barriers: availability of research and evaluation resources, resistance to rigorous evaluation, and convincing policy makers to use evaluation results (NASEM, 2017). These barriers, while important, are addressable, and AHRQ working with relevant government agencies and key stakeholders can develop programs to improve the evaluation of the effect of USPSTF guidelines.

COMMITTEE VISION

This committee approached the taxonomy and recommendations as an important component of a much larger effort for AHRQ, ODP, and USPSTF partners and other stakeholders to improve clinical prevention research and thereby practice. They may find success in this endeavor not only by implementing this committee's taxonomy and recommendations but also by adapting the committee's vision to improve clinical prevention research and practice in the United States. The committee acknowledges that to do so will increase the burden on ODP and NIH staff and the USPSTF members. Resources will be needed to accomplish this. The committee's vision (see Figure 5-1) comprises activities, outputs, and short-term and long-term outcomes.

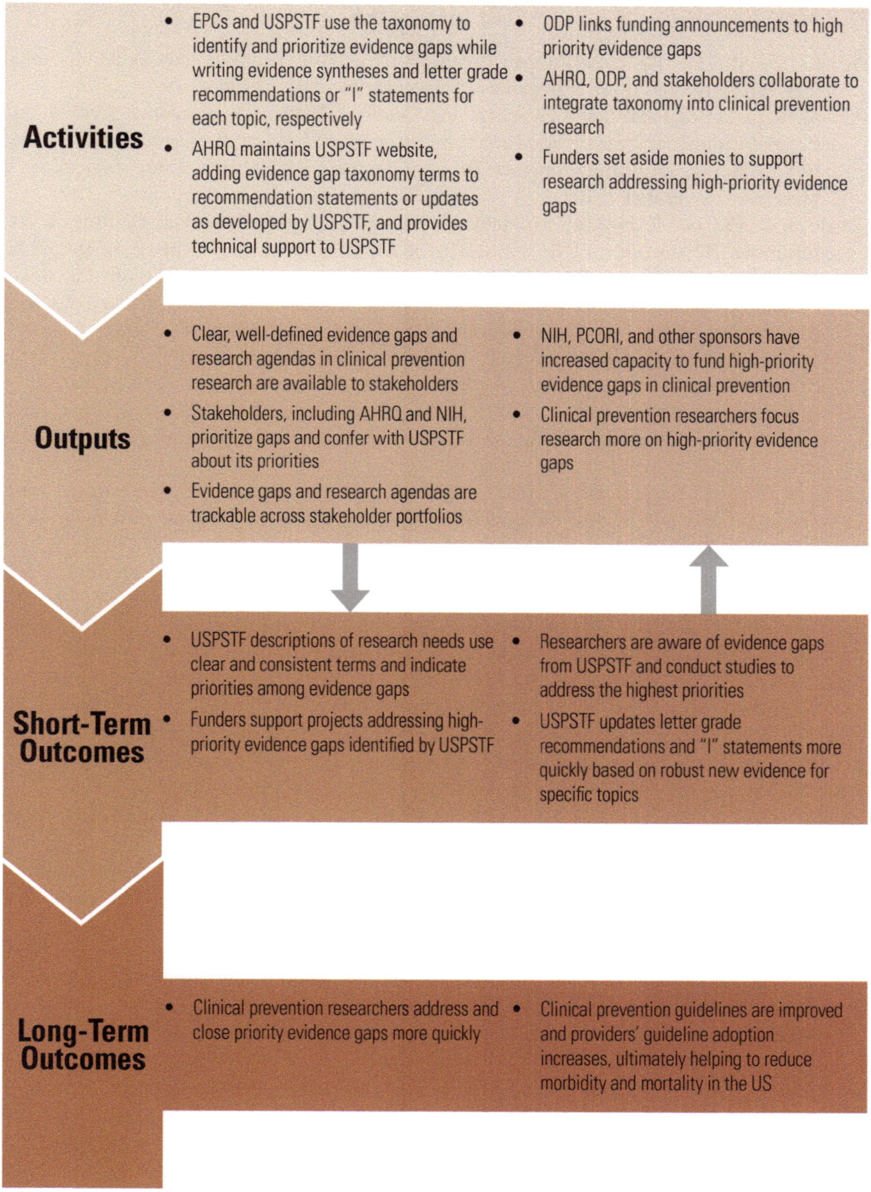

FIGURE 5-1 The committee vision for improving clinical prevention research.
NOTE: AHRQ = Agency for Healthcare Research and Quality; EPC = Evidence-based Practice Center; NIH = National Institutes of Health; ODP = Office of Disease Prevention; PCORI = Patient-Centered Outcomes Research Institute; USPSTF = U.S. Preventive Services Task Force.

REFERENCES

Adams, J., and S. Neville. 2020. Program evaluation for health professionals: What it is, what it isn't and how to do it. *International Journal of Qualitative Methods* 19.

AHRQ (Agency for Healthcare Research and Quality). 2018. *U.S. Preventive Services Task Force procedures for evidence-based practice centers.* https://www.ahrq.gov/sites/default/files/wysiwyg/funding/contracts/epc-vi/2-uspstf_procedures_guide_for_epcs.pdf (accessed November 3, 2021).

Cardoso, R., F. Guo., T. Heisser, M. Hackl, P. Ihle, H. De Schutter, N. Van Damme, Z. Valerianova, T. Atanasov, O. Májek, J. Mužík, M. C. Nilbert, A. J. Tybjerg, K. Innos, M. Mägi, N. Malila, A. M. Bouvier, V. Bouvier, G. Launoy, et al. 2021. Colorectal cancer incidence, mortality, and stage distribution in European countries in the colorectal cancer screening era: An international population-based study. *The Lancet Oncology* 22(7):P1002–P1013.

Davidson, K. W., A. H. Krist, C. Tseng, M. Simon, C. A. Doubeni, A. R. Kemper, M. Kubik, Q. Ngo-Metzger, J. Mills, and A. Borsky. 2021. Incorporation of social risk in US Preventive Services Task Force recommendations and identification of key challenges for primary care. *JAMA* 326(14):1410–1415.

Doubeni, C. A., M. Simon, and A. H. Krist. 2021. Addressing systemic racism through clinical preventive service recommendations from the US Preventive Services Task Force. *JAMA* 325(7):627–628.

Elliott, J. H., A. Synnot, T. Turner, M. Simmonds, E. A. Akl, S. McDonald, G. Salanti, J. Meerpohl, H. MacLehose, J. Hilton, D. Tovey, I. Shemilt, J. Thomas, and Living Systematic Review Network. 2017. Living systematic review: 1. Introduction—The why, what, when, and how. *Journal of Clinical Epidemiology* 91:23–30.

Frye, A. W., and P. A. Hemmer. 2012. Program evaluation models and related theories: AMEE guide no. 67. *Medical Teacher* 34(5):e288–e299.

Hall, I. J., F. K. Tangka, S. A. Sabatino, T. D. Thompson, B. I. Graubard, and N. Breen. 2018. Patterns and trends in cancer screening in the United States. *Preventing Chronic Disease* 15:170465.

Jonnalagadda, S. R., P. Goyal, and M. D. Huffman. 2015. Automating data extraction in systematic reviews: A systematic review. *Systematic Reviews* 4(78).

KFF (Kaiser Family Foundation). 2015. *Preventive services covered by private health plans under the Affordable Care Act.* https://www.kff.org/health-reform/fact-sheet/preventive-services-covered-by-private-health-plans (accessed July 19, 2021).

Klabunde, C. N., E. M. Ellis, J. Villani, E. Neilson, K. Schwartz, E. A. Vogt, and Q. Ngo-Metzger. 2021. Characteristics of scientific evidence informing changed U.S. Preventive Services Task Force insufficient evidence statements. *American Journal of Preventive Medicine*. https://www.sciencedirect.com/science/article/abs/pii/S0749379721004578 (accessed November 29, 2021).

Lau, J. 2019. Editorial: Systematic review automation thematic series. *Systematic Reviews* 8:70.

Mabry-Hernandez, I. R., S. J. Curry, W. R. Phillips, F. A. Garcia, K. W. Davidson, J. W. Epling, Jr., Q. Ngo-Metzger, and A. S. Bierman. 2018. U.S. Preventive Services Task Force priorities for prevention research. *American Journal of Preventive Medicine* 54(1 Suppl 1) S95–S103.

Manuel, L., L. S. Fong, T. Ly, and G. Meredith. 2021. Does lung cancer screening with low-dose computerized tomography improve survival? *Interactive Cardiovascular and Thoracic Surgery* ivab154.

Marshall, I. J., A. Noel-Storr, J. Kuiper, J. Thomas, and B. C. Wallace. 2018. Machine learning for identifying randomized controlled trials: An evaluation and practitioner's guide. *Research Synthesis Methods* 9(4):602–614.

McDonagh, M. S., J. Wagner, A. Y. Ahmed, B. Morasco, D. Kansagara and R. Chou. 2021. *Living systematic review on cannabis and other plant-based treatments for chronic pain—quarterly progress report.* Rockville, MD: Agency for Healthcare Research and Quality. https://doi.org/10.23970/AHRQEPCCER250.

Murad, M. H., S. M. Chang, C. Fiordalisi, J. S. Lin, T. J. Wilt, A. Tsou, B. Leas, S. Siddique, A. R. Zullo, E. Balk, C. M. Rutter, K. Robinson, C. Coleman, O. Costa, E. Stoeger, M. Helfand, and M. Viswanathan. 2021. Improving the utility of evidence synthesis for decision makers in the face of insufficient evidence. *AHRQ Methods for Effective Health Care.* https://www.ncbi.nlm.nih.gov/books/NBK569735 (accessed October 28, 2021).

Murray, D. M. 2017. Prevention research at the National Institutes of Health. *Public Health Reports* 132(5):535–538.

NASEM (National Academies of Sciences, Engineering, and Medicine). 2017. *Principles and practices for federal program evaluation: Proceedings of a workshop.* Washington, DC: The National Academies Press. https://doi.org/10.17226/24831.

NASEM. 2020. *Addressing evidence gaps in clinical prevention: Meeting 1.* 2nd Session. December 15, 2020, by the Committee on Addressing Evidence Gaps in Clinical Prevention Recommendations. https://www.nationalacademies.org/event/12-15-2020/addressing-evidence-gaps-in-clinical-prevention-committee-meeting-1-session-2 (accessed October 28, 2021).

NIH (National Institutes of Health). 2020. *What we do: Budget.* https://www.nih.gov/about-nih/what-we-do/budget (accessed August 10, 2021).

Rosenfeld, R. M., R. N. Shiffman, and P. Robertson. 2013. Clinical practice guideline development manual, third edition: A quality-driven approach for translating evidence into action. *Otolaryngology—Head and Neck Surgery* 148:S1–S55.

USPSTF (U.S. Preventive Services Task Force). 2011. *First annual report to Congress on high-priority evidence gaps for clinical preventive services.* https://www.uspreventiveservicestaskforce.org/uspstf/about-uspstf/reports-congress/first-annual-report-congress-high-priority-evidence-gaps-clinical-preventive-services (accessed August 27, 2021).

USPSTF. 2017. *Celiac disease: Screening.* https://www.uspreventiveservicestaskforce.org/uspstf/recommendation/celiac-disease-screening (accessed August 17, 2021).

USPSTF. 2018a. *Cardiovascular disease: Risk assessment with nontraditional risk factors.* https://www.uspreventiveservicestaskforce.org/uspstf/recommendation/cardiovascular-disease-screening-using-nontraditional-risk-assessment (accessed August 17, 2021).

USPSTF. 2018b. *Child maltreatment: Interventions.* https://www.uspreventiveservicestaskforce.org/uspstf/recommendation/child-maltreatment-primary-care-interventions (accessed August 17, 2021).

USPSTF. 2018c. *Intimate partner violence, elder abuse, and abuse of vulnerable adults: Screening.* https://www.uspreventiveservicestaskforce.org/uspstf/recommendation/intimate-partner-violence-and-abuse-of-elderly-and-vulnerable-adults-screening (accessed August 17, 2021).

USPSTF. 2019. *Abdominal aortic aneurysm: Screening.* https://www.uspreventiveservicestaskforce.org/uspstf/recommendation/abdominal-aortic-aneurysm-screening (accessed August 17, 2021).

USPSTF. 2020. *Illicit drug use in children, adolescents, and young adults: Primary care-based interventions.* https://www.uspreventiveservicestaskforce.org/uspstf/recommendation/drug-use-illicit-primary-care-interventions-for-children-and-adolescents (accessed August 17, 2021).

USPSTF. 2021a. *Chlamydia and gonnorhea: Screening.* https://www.uspreventiveservicestaskforce.org/uspstf/recommendation/chlamydia-and-gonorrhea-screening (accessed November 3, 2021).

USPSTF. 2021b. *Gestational diabetes: Screening*. https://www.uspreventiveservicestaskforce.org/uspstf/recommendation/gestational-diabetes-screening (accessed August 17, 2021).

USPSTF. 2021c. *Lung cancer: Screening*. https://www.uspreventiveservicestaskforce.org/uspstf/recommendation/lung-cancer-screening (accessed November 3, 2021).

USPSTF. 2021d. *Tobacco smoking cessation in adults, including pregnant persons: Interventions*. https://www.uspreventiveservicestaskforce.org/uspstf/recommendation/tobacco-use-in-adults-and-pregnant-women-counseling-and-interventions (accessed August 17, 2021).

A

Topics with "I Statements" from the U.S. Preventive Services Task Force

This appendix contains a summary table (see Table A-1) of all topics addressed by the U.S. Preventive Services Task Force (USPSTF) that include an "I statement" for at least one recommendation regarding the topic. Some topics have only one grade (e.g., screening for hearing loss in older adults), while some have multiple "I statements" along with letter grade recommendations for different aspects of a preventive service (e.g., screening for breast cancer), and still others have a letter grade for one group and an "I statement" for another group (e.g., screening for unhealthy drug use).

TABLE A-1 Topics with "I Statements" from the U.S. Preventive Services Task Force

Topic Name	Year	Grade	Specific Recommendation
Chlamydia and Gonorrhea: Screening[1]	2021	B	The USPSTF recommends screening for chlamydia in sexually active women age 24 years and younger and in older women who are at increased risk for infection.
		B	The USPSTF recommends screening for gonorrhea in sexually active women age 24 years and younger and in older women who are at increased risk for infection.
		I	The USPSTF concludes that the current evidence is insufficient to assess the balance of benefits and harms of screening for chlamydia and gonorrhea in men.
Gestational Diabetes: Screening[2]	2021	B	Asymptomatic pregnant persons at 24 weeks of gestation or after
		I	Asymptomatic pregnant persons before 24 weeks of gestation
Vitamin D Deficiency in Adults: Screening[3]	2021	I	
Hearing Loss in Older Adults: Screening[4]	2021	I	

[1] USPSTF, 2021a.
[2] USPSTF, 2021b.
[3] USPSTF, 2021e.
[4] USPSTF, 2021c.

TABLE A-1 Continued

Tobacco Smoking Cessation in Adults, Including Pregnant Persons: Interventions[5]	2021	A	The USPSTF recommends that clinicians ask all adults about tobacco use, advise them to stop using tobacco, and provide behavioral interventions and U.S. Food and Drug Administration (FDA)-approved pharmacotherapy for cessation to nonpregnant adults who use tobacco.
		A	The USPSTF recommends that clinicians ask all pregnant persons about tobacco use, advise them to stop using tobacco, and provide behavioral interventions for cessation to pregnant persons who use tobacco.
		I	The USPSTF concludes that the current evidence is insufficient to assess the balance of benefits and harms of pharmacotherapy interventions for tobacco cessation in pregnant persons.
		I	The USPSTF concludes that the current evidence is insufficient to assess the balance of benefits and harms of electronic cigarettes (e-cigarettes) for tobacco cessation in adults, including pregnant persons. The USPSTF recommends that clinicians direct patients who use tobacco to other tobacco cessation interventions with proven effectiveness and established safety. See the Practice Considerations section for more information on recommended behavioral interventions and pharmacotherapy and for suggestions for practice regarding the I statements.
High Blood Pressure in Children and Adolescents: Screening[6]	2020	I	
Unhealthy Drug Use: Screening[7]	2020	B	Adults aged 18 and older
		I	Adolescents
Illicit Drug Use in Children, Adolescents, and Young Adults: Primary Care–Based Interventions[8]	2020	I	

[5] USPSTF, 2021d.
[6] USPSTF, 2020c.
[7] USPSTF, 2020f.
[8] USPSTF, 2020d.

TABLE A-1 Continued

Tobacco Use in Children and Adolescents: Primary Care Interventions[9]	2020	B	School-aged children and adolescents who have not started to use tobacco
		I	School-aged children and adolescents who use tobacco
Bacterial Vaginosis in Pregnant Persons to Prevent Preterm Delivery: Screening[10]	2020	D	Pregnant persons not at increased risk for preterm delivery
		I	Pregnant persons at increased risk for preterm delivery
Cognitive Impairment in Older Adults: Screening[11]	2020	I	
Abdominal Aortic Aneurysm: Screening[12]	2019	B	The USPSTF recommends 1-time screening for abdominal aortic aneurysm (AAA) with ultrasonography in men aged 65 to 75 years who have ever smoked.
		C	The USPSTF recommends that clinicians selectively offer screening for AAA with ultrasonography in men aged 65–75 years who have never smoked rather than routinely screening all men in this group. Evidence indicates that the net benefit of screening all men in this group is small. In determining whether this service is appropriate in individual cases, patients and clinicians should consider the balance of benefits and harms on the basis of evidence relevant to the patient's medical history, family history, other risk factors, and personal values.
		D	The USPSTF recommends against routine screening for AAA with ultrasonography in women who have never smoked and have no family history of AAA.
		I	The USPSTF concludes that the current evidence is insufficient to assess the balance of benefits and harms of screening for AAA with ultrasonography in women aged 65–75 years who have ever smoked or have a family history of AAA.

[9] USPSTF, 2020e.
[10] USPSTF, 2020a.
[11] USPSTF, 2020b.
[12] USPSTF, 2019a.

TABLE A-1 Continued

Elevated Blood Lead Levels in Children and Pregnant Women: Screening[13]	2019	I	The USPSTF concludes that the current evidence is insufficient to assess the balance of benefits and harms of screening for elevated blood lead levels in asymptomatic pregnant persons.
		I	The USPSTF concludes that the current evidence is insufficient to assess the balance of benefits and harms of screening for elevated blood lead levels in asymptomatic children.
Child Maltreatment: Interventions[14]	2018	I	
Unhealthy Alcohol Use in Adolescents and Adults: Screening and Behavioral Counseling Interventions[15]	2018	B	Adults 18 years or older, including pregnant women
		I	Adolescents aged 12–17 years
Intimate Partner Violence, Elder Abuse, and Abuse of Vulnerable Adults: Screening[16]	2018	B	Women of reproductive age
		I	Older or vulnerable adults
Atrial Fibrillation: Screening with Electrocardiography[17]	2018	I	
Peripheral Artery Disease and Cardiovascular Disease: Screening and Risk Assessment with the Ankle-Brachial Index[18]	2018	I	
Cardiovascular Disease: Risk Assessment with Nontraditional Risk Factors[19]	2018	I	

[13] USPSTF, 2019b.
[14] USPSTF, 2018e.
[15] USPSTF, 2018j.
[16] USPSTF, 2018f.
[17] USPSTF, 2018b.
[18] USPSTF, 2018h.
[19] USPSTF, 2018d.

TABLE A-1 Continued

Osteoporosis to Prevent Fractures: Screening[20]	2018	B	Women 65 years and older
		B	Postmenopausal women younger than 65 years at increased risk of osteoporosis
		I	Men
Cardiovascular Disease Risk: Screening with Electrocardiography[21]	2018	D	Adults at low risk of cardiovascular disease (CVD) events
		I	Adults at intermediate or high risk of CVD events
Vitamin D, Calcium, or Combined Supplementation for the Primary Prevention of Fractures in Community-Dwelling Adults: Preventive Medication[22]	2018	D	The USPSTF recommends against daily supplementation with 400 IU or less of vitamin D and 1,000 mg or less of calcium for the primary prevention of fractures in community-dwelling, postmenopausal women.
		I	The USPSTF concludes that the current evidence is insufficient to assess the balance of the benefits and harms of vitamin D and calcium supplementation, alone or combined, for the primary prevention of fractures in men and premenopausal women.
		I	The USPSTF concludes that the current evidence is insufficient to assess the balance of the benefits and harms of daily supplementation with doses greater than 400 IU of vitamin D and greater than 1000 mg of calcium for the primary prevention of fractures in community-dwelling, postmenopausal women.
Skin Cancer Prevention: Behavioral Counseling[23]	2018	B	Young adults, adolescents, children, and parents of young children
		C	Adults older than 24 years with fair skin types
		I	Adults
Adolescent Idiopathic Scoliosis: Screening[24]	2018	I	

[20] USPSTF, 2018g.
[21] USPSTF, 2018c.
[22] USPSTF, 2018k.
[23] USPSTF, 2018i.
[24] USPSTF, 2018a.

TABLE A-1 Continued

Vision in Children Ages 6 Months to 5 Years: Screening[25]	2017	B	Children aged 3–5 years
		I	Children younger than 3 years
Celiac Disease: Screening[26]	2017	I	
Gynecological Conditions: Periodic Screening with the Pelvic Examination[27]	2017	I	
Obstructive Sleep Apnea in Adults: Screening[28]	2017	I	
Statin Use for the Primary Prevention of Cardiovascular Disease in Adults: Preventive Medication[29]	2016	B	Adults aged 40 to 75 years with no history of CVD, 1 or more CVD risk factors, and a calculated 10-year CVD event risk of 10% or greater
		C	Adults aged 40 to 75 years with no history of CVD, 1 or more CVD risk factors, and a calculated 10-year CVD event risk of 7.5% to 10%
		I	Adults 76 years and older with no history of CVD
Lipid Disorders in Children and Adolescents: Screening[30]	2016	I	
Skin Cancer: Screening[31]	2016	I	
Aspirin Use to Prevent Cardiovascular Disease and Colorectal Cancer: Preventive Medication[32]	2016	B	Adults aged 50–59 years with a 10% or greater 10-year CVD risk
		C	Adults aged 60–69 years with a 10% or greater 10-year CVD risk
		I	Adults younger than 50 years
		I	Adults aged 70 or older

[25] USPSTF, 2017d.
[26] USPSTF, 2017a.
[27] USPSTF, 2017b.
[28] USPSTF, 2017c.
[29] USPSTF, 2016h.
[30] USPSTF, 2016f.
[31] USPSTF, 2016g.
[32] USPSTF, 2016a.

TABLE A-1 Continued

Impaired Visual Acuity in Older Adults: Screening[33]	2016	I	
Autism Spectrum Disorder in Young Children: Screening[34]	2016	I	
Depression in Children and Adolescents: Screening[35]	2016	B	Adolescents aged 12–18 years
	2016	I	Children aged 11 years or younger
Breast Cancer: Screening[36]	2016	B	Women aged 50–74 years
		C	Women aged 40–49 years
		I	All women
		I	Women with dense breasts
		I	Women aged 75 years or older
Iron Deficiency Anemia in Young Children: Screening[37]	2015	I	
Iron Deficiency Anemia in Pregnant Women: Screening and Supplementation[38]	2015	I	
Speech and Language Delay and Disorders in Children Age 5 and Younger: Screening[39]	2015	I	
Thyroid Dysfunction: Screening[40]	2015	I	
Suicide Risk in Adolescents, Adults, and Older Adults: Screening[41]	2014	I	

[33] USPSTF, 2016e.
[34] USPSTF, 2016b.
[35] USPSTF, 2016d.
[36] USPSTF, 2016c.
[37] USPSTF, 2015b.
[38] USPSTF, 2015a.
[39] USPSTF, 2015c.
[40] USPSTF, 2015d.
[41] USPSTF, 2014b.

TABLE A-1 Continued

Dental Caries in Children from Birth Through Age 5 Years: Screening[42]	2014	B	Children from Birth Through Age 5 Years: The USPSTF recommends that primary care clinicians prescribe oral fluoride supplementation starting at age 6 months for children whose water supply is deficient in fluoride.
		B	Children from Birth Through Age 5 Years: The USPSTF recommends that primary care clinicians apply fluoride varnish to the primary teeth of all infants and children starting at the age of primary tooth eruption.
		I	Children from Birth Through Age 5 Years: The USPSTF concludes that the current evidence is insufficient to assess the balance of benefits and harms of routine screening examinations for dental caries performed by primary care clinicians in children from birth to age 5 years.
Vitamin Supplementation to Prevent Cancer and CVD: Preventive Medication[43]	2014	D	The USPSTF recommends against the use of ß-carotene or vitamin E supplements for the prevention of cardiovascular disease or cancer.
		I	The USPSTF concludes that the current evidence is insufficient to assess the balance of benefits and harms of the use of multivitamins for the prevention of cardiovascular disease or cancer.
		I	The USPSTF concludes that the current evidence is insufficient to assess the balance of benefits and harms of the use of single- or paired-nutrient supplements (except ß-carotene and vitamin E) for the prevention of cardiovascular disease or cancer.
Oral Cancer: Screening[44]	2013	I	
Glaucoma: Screening[45]	2013	I	
Bladder Cancer in Adults: Screening[46]	2011	I	

[42] USPSTF, 2014a.
[43] USPSTF, 2014c.
[44] USPSTF, 2013b.
[45] USPSTF, 2013a.
[46] USPSTF, 2011.

REFERENCES

USPSTF (U.S. Preventive Services Task Force). 2011. *Bladder cancer in adults: Screening.* https://www.uspreventiveservicestaskforce.org/uspstf/recommendation/bladder-cancer-in-adults-screening (accessed August 17, 2021).

USPSTF. 2013a. *Glaucoma: Screening.* https://www.uspreventiveservicestaskforce.org/uspstf/recommendation/glaucoma-screening (accessed August 17, 2021).

USPSTF. 2013b. *Oral cancer: Screening.* https://www.uspreventiveservicestaskforce.org/uspstf/recommendation/oral-cancer-screening (accessed August 17, 2021).

USPSTF. 2014a. *Dental caries in children from birth through age 5 years: Screening.* https://www.uspreventiveservicestaskforce.org/uspstf/recommendation/dental-caries-in-children-from-birth-through-age-5-years-screening (accessed August 17, 2021).

USPSTF. 2014b. *Suicide risk in adolescents, adults and older adults: Screening.* https://www.uspreventiveservicestaskforce.org/uspstf/recommendation/suicide-risk-in-adolescents-adults-and-older-adults-screening (accessed August 17, 2021).

USPSTF. 2014c. *Vitamin supplementation to prevent cancer and CVD: Preventive medication.* https://www.uspreventiveservicestaskforce.org/uspstf/recommendation/vitamin-supplementation-to-prevent-cancer-and-cvd-counseling (accessed August 17, 2021).

USPSTF. 2015a. *Iron deficiency anemia in pregnant women: Screening and supplementation.* https://www.uspreventiveservicestaskforce.org/uspstf/recommendation/iron-deficiency-anemia-in-pregnant-women-screening-and-supplementation (accessed August 17, 2021).

USPSTF. 2015b. *Iron deficiency anemia in young children: Screening.* https://www.uspreventiveservicestaskforce.org/uspstf/recommendation/iron-deficiency-anemia-in-young-children-screening (accessed August 17, 2021).

USPSTF. 2015c. *Speech and language delay and disorders in children age 5 and younger: Screening.* https://www.uspreventiveservicestaskforce.org/uspstf/recommendation/speech-and-language-delay-and-disorders-in-children-age-5-and-younger-screening (accessed August 17, 2021).

USPSTF. 2015d. *Thyroid dysfunction: Screening.* https://www.uspreventiveservicestaskforce.org/uspstf/recommendation/thyroid-dysfunction-screening (accessed August 17, 2021).

USPSTF. 2016a. *Aspirin use to prevent cardiovascular disease and colorectal cancer: Preventive medication.* https://www.uspreventiveservicestaskforce.org/uspstf/recommendation/aspirin-to-prevent-cardiovascular-disease-and-cancer (accessed August 17, 2021).

USPSTF. 2016b. *Autism spectrum disorder in young children: Screening.* https://www.uspreventiveservicestaskforce.org/uspstf/recommendation/autism-spectrum-disorder-in-young-children-screening (accessed August 17, 2021).

USPSTF. 2016c. *Breast cancer: Screening.* https://www.uspreventiveservicestaskforce.org/uspstf/recommendation/breast-cancer-screening (accessed August 17, 2021).

USPSTF. 2016d. *Depression in children and adolescents: Screening.* https://www.uspreventiveservicestaskforce.org/uspstf/recommendation/depression-in-children-and-adolescents-screening (accessed August 17, 2021).

USPSTF. 2016e. *Impaired visual activity in older adults: Screening.* https://www.uspreventiveservicestaskforce.org/uspstf/recommendation/impaired-visual-acuity-in-older-adults-screening (accessed August 17, 2021).

USPSTF. 2016f. *Lipid disorders in children and adolescents: Screening.* https://www.uspreventiveservicestaskforce.org/uspstf/recommendation/lipid-disorders-in-children-screening (accessed August 17, 2021).

USPSTF. 2016g. *Skin cancer: Screening.* https://www.uspreventiveservicestaskforce.org/uspstf/recommendation/skin-cancer-screening (accessed August 17, 2021).

USPSTF. 2016h. *Statin use for the primary prevention of cardiovascular disease in adults: Preventive medication*. https://www.uspreventiveservicestaskforce.org/uspstf/recommendation/statin-use-in-adults-preventive-medication (accessed August 17, 2021).

USPSTF. 2017a. *Celiac disease: Screening*. https://www.uspreventiveservicestaskforce.org/uspstf/recommendation/celiac-disease-screening (accessed August 17, 2021).

USPSTF. 2017b. *Gynecological conditions: Periodic screening with the pelvic examination*. https://www.uspreventiveservicestaskforce.org/uspstf/recommendation/gynecological-conditions-screening-with-the-pelvic-examination (accessed August 17, 2021).

USPSTF. 2017c. *Obstructive sleep apnea in adults: Screening*. https://www.uspreventiveservicestaskforce.org/uspstf/recommendation/obstructive-sleep-apnea-in-adults-screening (accessed August 17, 2021).

USPSTF. 2017d. *Vision in children ages 6 months to 5 years: Screening*. https://www.uspreventiveservicestaskforce.org/uspstf/recommendation/vision-in-children-ages-6-months-to-5-years-screening (accessed August 17, 2021).

USPSTF. 2018a. *Adolescent idiopathic scoliosis: Screening*. https://www.uspreventiveservicestaskforce.org/uspstf/recommendation/adolescent-idiopathic-scoliosis-screening (accessed August 17, 2021).

USPSTF. 2018b. *Atrial fibrillation: Screening with electrocardiography*. https://www.uspreventiveservicestaskforce.org/uspstf/recommendation/atrial-fibrillation-screening-with-electrocardiography (accessed August 17, 2021).

USPSTF. 2018c. *Cardiovascular disease risk: Screening with electrocardiography*. https://www.uspreventiveservicestaskforce.org/uspstf/recommendation/cardiovascular-disease-risk-screening-with-electrocardiography (accessed August 17, 2021).

USPSTF. 2018d. *Cardiovascular disease: Risk assessment with nontraditional risk factors*. https://www.uspreventiveservicestaskforce.org/uspstf/recommendation/cardiovascular-disease-screening-using-nontraditional-risk-assessment (accessed August 17, 2021).

USPSTF. 2018e. *Child maltreatment: Interventions*. https://www.uspreventiveservicestaskforce.org/uspstf/recommendation/child-maltreatment-primary-care-interventions (accessed August 17, 2021).

USPSTF. 2018f. *Intimate partner violence, elder abuse, and abuse of vulnerable adults: Screening*. https://www.uspreventiveservicestaskforce.org/uspstf/recommendation/intimate-partner-violence-and-abuse-of-elderly-and-vulnerable-adults-screening (accessed August 17, 2021).

USPSTF. 2018g. *Osteoporosis to prevent fractures: Screening*. https://www.uspreventiveservicestaskforce.org/uspstf/recommendation/osteoporosis-screening (accessed August 17, 2021).

USPSTF. 2018h. *Peripheral artery disease and cardiovascular disease: Screening and risk assessment with the ankle-brachial index*. https://www.uspreventiveservicestaskforce.org/uspstf/recommendation/peripheral-artery-disease-in-adults-screening-with-the-ankle-brachial-index (accessed August 17, 2021).

USPSTF. 2018i. *Skin cancer prevention: Behavioral counseling*. https://www.uspreventiveservicestaskforce.org/uspstf/recommendation/skin-cancer-counseling (accessed August 17, 2021).

USPSTF. 2018j. *Unhealthy alcohol use in adolescents and adults: Screening and behavioral counseling interventions*. https://www.uspreventiveservicestaskforce.org/uspstf/recommendation/unhealthy-alcohol-use-in-adolescents-and-adults-screening-and-behavioral-counseling-interventions (accessed August 17, 2021).

USPSTF. 2018k. *Vitamin D, calcium, or combined supplementation for the primary prevention of fractures in community-dwelling adults: Preventive medication*. https://www.uspreventiveservicestaskforce.org/uspstf/recommendation/vitamin-d-calcium-or-combined-supplementation-for-the-primary-prevention-of-fractures-in-adults-preventive-medication (accessed August 17, 2021).

USPSTF. 2019a. *Abdominal aortic aneurysm: Screening*. https://www.uspreventiveservicestaskforce.org/uspstf/recommendation/abdominal-aortic-aneurysm-screening (accessed August 17, 2021).

USPSTF. 2019b. *Elevated blood lead levels in children and pregnant women: Screening*. https://www.uspreventiveservicestaskforce.org/uspstf/recommendation/elevated-blood-lead-levels-in-childhood-and-pregnancy-screening (accessed August 17, 2021).

USPSTF. 2020a. *Bacterial vaginosis in pregnant persons to prevent preterm delivery: Screening*. https://www.uspreventiveservicestaskforce.org/uspstf/recommendation/bacterial-vaginosis-in-pregnancy-to-prevent-preterm-delivery-screening (accessed August 17, 2021).

USPSTF. 2020b. *Cognitive impairment in older adults: Screening*. https://www.uspreventiveservicestaskforce.org/uspstf/recommendation/cognitive-impairment-in-older-adults-screening (accessed August 17, 2021).

USPSTF. 2020c. *High blood pressure in children and adolescents: Screening*. https://www.uspreventiveservicestaskforce.org/uspstf/recommendation/blood-pressure-in-children-and-adolescents-hypertension-screening (accessed August 17, 2021).

USPSTF. 2020d. *Illicit drug use in children, adolescents, and young adults: Primary care-based interventions*. https://www.uspreventiveservicestaskforce.org/uspstf/recommendation/drug-use-illicit-primary-care-interventions-for-children-and-adolescents (accessed August 17, 2021).

USPSTF. 2020e. *Tobacco use in children and adolescents: Primary care interventions*. https://www.uspreventiveservicestaskforce.org/uspstf/recommendation/tobacco-and-nicotine-use-prevention-in-children-and-adolescents-primary-care-interventions (accessed August 17, 2021).

USPSTF. 2020f. *Unhealthy drug use: Screening*. https://www.uspreventiveservicestaskforce.org/uspstf/recommendation/drug-use-illicit-screening (accessed August 17, 2021).

USPSTF. 2021a. *Chlamydia and gonorrhea: Screening*. https://www.uspreventiveservicestaskforce.org/uspstf/recommendation/chlamydia-and-gonorrhea-screening (accessed August 17, 2021).

USPSTF. 2021b. *Gestational diabetes: Screening*. https://www.uspreventiveservicestaskforce.org/uspstf/recommendation/gestational-diabetes-screening (accessed August 17, 2021).

USPSTF. 2021c. *Hearing loss in older adults: Screening*. https://www.uspreventiveservicestaskforce.org/uspstf/recommendation/hearing-loss-in-older-adults-screening (accessed August 17, 2021).

USPSTF. 2021d. *Tobacco smoking cessation in adults, including pregnant persons: Interventions*. https://www.uspreventiveservicestaskforce.org/uspstf/recommendation/tobacco-use-in-adults-and-pregnant-women-counseling-and-interventions (accessed August 17, 2021).

USPSTF. 2021e. *Vitamin D deficiency in adults: Screening*. https://www.uspreventiveservicestaskforce.org/uspstf/recommendation/vitamin-d-deficiency-screening (accessed August 17, 2021).

B

Research Methods

Evaluating the quality of evidence for key questions on the benefits and harms of preventive services forms a cornerstone of the U.S. Preventive Services Task Force (USPSTF) and the Community Preventive Services Task Force processes. Researchers who produce this evidence often face tradeoffs among an array of possible study designs that can be used for research on whether an action (e.g., screening, behavioral counseling, or preventive medication) causes an outcome. Randomized controlled trials (RCTs) are widely considered to produce the highest-quality evidence because they are less prone to confounding than observational study designs. However, evidence from RCTs often has key limitations in generalizability to real-life populations and settings.

New designs for RCTs and innovative methods for observational studies have gained increasing traction in health care delivery research in the past two decades. Modern study designs could enable researchers to address evidence gaps in the USPSTF analytic framework where traditional individual-level RCTs are not feasible for a variety of reasons. In addition, innovative designs can be useful for studies to address gaps in the research foundation, and in real-world dissemination and implementation of recommended preventive services. In this chapter, the committee discusses the types of studies needed to fill different types of evidence gaps, considering both existing USPSTF methods and innovative modern methods. Our purpose is to highlight specific newer study designs particularly germane to clinical prevention research, and to encourage researchers, sponsors, and guideline committees to increase their use and acceptance where appropriate.

TYPES OF STUDIES NEEDED TO FILL EVIDENCE GAPS

To identify the types of studies needed to fill evidence gaps for recent USPSTF-reviewed topics, the committee evaluated all "Research Needs and Gaps" sections from all 14 USPSTF recommendations that contained any "insufficient evidence" (I) statement published over 3 years, from July 2018 to June 2021. Five of these 14 statements contained I statements along with letter grade recommendations (A, B, C, or D) for part of the population or intervention, with the I statement applying to a subgroup or to a specific type of intervention. The committee also reviewed all nine statements containing only A, B, C, or D grades published from January 2020 to June 2021.

Among the 14 USPSTF recommendations reviewed containing an I statement, four specifically called for RCTs (see Table B-1). Others called for evidence about the effectiveness of screening or intervention without specifying a required study design. Ten of the 14 called for studies of risk prediction approaches (i.e., ways to identify high-risk groups). Of these, several statements requested research on how high-risk subgroups could be identified using clinical information such as data from questionnaires. Others requested research to establish the best specifications for a physical test, such as determining the preferred laboratory test for vitamin D deficiency, or developing consistent definitions of hearing loss to improve certainty about the accuracy of screening tests. Five of the 14 recommendations described evidence gaps that would require longitudinal follow-up of patients, either in RCTs or cohort studies, such as understanding the long-term history of hypertension in children and how often it resolves spontaneously. Half of the statements called for more research on population subgroups defined by age, sex, race or ethnicity, or other factors. Three requested research on real-world dissemination or implementation. One statement, on abdominal aortic aneurysm screening, suggested that high-quality modeling studies for women could be informative if new trials were not available.

Of the nine USPSTF recommendations reviewed containing letter grades and no I statements, six specifically requested additional RCTs. Seven called for studies of risk prediction approaches, and six requested studies to refine the specifications of the intervention or to test related new interventions. Three described research needs that could best be met by longitudinal cohort studies or trials with long-term follow-up. Two mentioned research needs related to dissemination and implementation.

TABLE B-1 Types of Studies Needed to Address Research Needs and Gaps Described in Recent U.S. Preventive Services Task Force Statements

	Study Type Specified or Implied in the Research Needs Section of the USPSTF Statement							
Topic	Randomized controlled trial (RCT)*	Intervention effectiveness study, unspecified*	Risk prediction study, including test performance	Longitudinal follow-up (in RCT or cohort study)	Cross-sectional study	Research in subgroups	Dissemination or Implementation study	Notes
Part 1. Recommendations containing an "insufficient evidence" (I) statement, July 2018–June 2021								
Vitamin D Deficiency in Adults: Screening		1	1					
Tobacco Smoking Cessation in Adults, Including Pregnant Persons: Interventions	1	1		1	1			Calls for studies of additional outcomes
Hearing Loss in Older Adults: Screening		1	1			1		

continued

TABLE B-1 Continued

	Study Type Specified or Implied in the Research Needs Section of the USPSTF Statement							
Topic	Randomized controlled trial (RCT)*	Intervention effectiveness study, unspecified*	Risk prediction study, including test performance	Longitudinal follow-up (in RCT or cohort study)	Cross-sectional study	Research in subgroups	Dissemination or Implementation study	Notes
High Blood Pressure in Children and Adolescents: Screening		1	1	1		1		RCTs could be difficult because this screening is routine in usual care
Prevention and Cessation of Tobacco Use in Children and Adolescents: Primary Care Interventions		1				1		
Unhealthy Drug Use: Screening		1	1				1	
Illicit Drug Use in Children, Adolescents, and Young Adults: Primary Care–Based Interventions		1				1	1	
Bacterial Vaginosis in Pregnant Persons to Prevent Preterm Delivery: Screening		1				1		

Cognitive Impairment in Older Adults: Screening		1	1					Calls for more consistent definitions of outcomes
Abdominal Aortic Aneurysm: Screening	1		1	1	1	1	1	Suggested high-quality modeling studies could be useful
Elevated Blood Lead Levels in Children and Pregnant Women: Screening		1	1	1				RCTs could be difficult because this screening is routine in usual care
Atrial Fibrillation: Screening with Electrocardiography	1		1					Mentions ongoing RCTs
Peripheral Artery Disease and Cardiovascular Disease: Screening and Risk Assessment with the Ankle-Brachial Index	1		1			1		Mentions ongoing RCTs
Cardiovascular Disease: Risk Assessment with Nontraditional Risk Factors		1	1	1			1	Requests studies of incremental benefit in real-world practice
Total	4	11	10	5	2	7	3	

continued

TABLE B-1 Continued

	Study Type Specified or Implied in the Research Needs Section of the USPSTF Statement							
Topic	Randomized controlled trial (RCT)*	Intervention effectiveness study, unspecified*	Risk prediction study, including test performance	Longitudinal follow-up (in RCT or cohort study)	Cross-sectional study	Research in subgroups	Dissemination or Implementation study	Notes
Part 2. Recommendations containing only A, B, C, or D grades								
Healthy Weight and Weight Gain in Pregnancy: Behavioral Counseling Interventions		1		1		1		
Colorectal Cancer: Screening	1	1	1			1	1	
Hypertension in Adults: Screening			1	1				

Lung Cancer: Screening			1				1	Requests studies of risk prediction models to select patients to screen
Asymptomatic Carotid Artery Stenosis: Screening	1		1					
Hepatitis B Virus Infection in Adolescents and Adults: Screening	1	1	1	1			1	Requests studies of decision support tools
Healthy Diet and Physical Activity for Cardiovascular Disease Prevention in Adults with Cardiovascular Risk Factors: Behavioral Counseling	1	1						
Sexually Transmitted Infections: Behavioral Counseling	1	1	1	1				
Hepatitis C Virus Infection in Adolescents and Adults: Screening	1	1	1			1		
Total	6	6	7	3	0	3	2	

* The Randomized Controlled Trial column was marked only when a Research Needs statement specified a randomized controlled trial. Other statements calling for research on the benefits of a screening, treatment, or other intervention were classified as "Intervention Effectiveness Study, unspecified."

PRODUCING HIGH-QUALITY EVIDENCE

The USPSTF rates the body of evidence for each question in the analytic framework for a given topic as convincing, adequate, or inadequate based on several factor (USPSTF, 2021). First among these is, "Do the studies have the appropriate research design to answer the key question(s)?" Other key factors considered in evaluating the adequacy of evidence include the internal validity and external generalizability to the U.S. primary care population, aggregated across all studies across each of the key questions.

The Grading of Recommendations Assessment, Development, and Evaluation (GRADE) system, introduced in 2011 based on the work of an international consensus group, is a widely used body of standards for rating the quality of a body of evidence in systematic reviews and guidelines for clinical, public health, and health systems questions. In the GRADE approach, RCTs are initially classified as high-quality evidence and observational studies as low-quality evidence for estimates of intervention effects (Guyatt et al., 2011). From these starting points, a body of evidence about whether an action (e.g., screening or treatment) causes an outcome may be downgraded or upgraded. Reasons for downgrading include bias, inconsistency, indirectness, imprecision, and publication bias. Reasons for upgrading include evidence of a large effect, a dose-response effect, and all plausible confounding would bias in the direction opposite of the observed effect (or lack of effect).

In recent years, GRADE guidance has been updated to suggest that the evaluation of non-randomized studies of interventions could begin with an assumption of high certainty with the use of a new tool called the Risk of Bias in Non-Randomized Studies of Interventions (ROBINS-I) (Schünemann et al., 2019; Sterne et al., 2016). The ROBINS-I tool enables reviewers to evaluate the risk of bias in estimates of comparative effectiveness (harm or benefit) in non-randomized studies of interventions and to assess the magnitude of bias in different domains, including confounding, selection, misclassification of intervention status, deviations from intended interventions, missing data, outcomes measurement, and reporting.

SELECTION OF STUDY DESIGNS

For many of the USPSTF recommendations reviewed in Table 5-1, it would be possible to address a research need using either an RCT or an observational study design. Many factors influence the selection of a study design by a sponsor or a researcher. These include the anticipated internal and external validity of the study design, and extrinsic factors including time urgency and logistical barriers (Armstrong, 2012). In addition, studies designed for diverse populations may also need to consider the possibility that the intervention may have heterogeneous effects on different subpopulations. Study designs that have high per-patient costs may lead to limited sample sizes and inadequate power to identify heterogeneity of treatment effect, making study designs with lower per-patient costs more attractive if they are of adequate quality.

Limitations of Individual-Level Randomized Controlled Trials

RCTs are not practically feasible or are not the optimal approach in some situations. Examples include preventive services where:

- The service is already widely accepted as standard of practice, such as lead screening for children. It would be difficult on ethical grounds to withhold standard care for a trial.
- The service would likely be viewed as desirable by the average patient, which could hinder enrolling a representative group in an individual-level trial.
- The service already has high-quality evidence for effectiveness in one patient group, and this evidence could be extrapolated to other patient groups. For example, abdominal aortic screening is recommended for men aged 65–75 years who have ever smoked. Given this, it could be argued that a similar trial of women of similar age and smoking history is not required.
- The cost and/or burden of enrolling patients individually precludes sponsors or clinicians from supporting a trial.

Individual-level RCTs have other important limitations. The results are often not externally generalizable because inclusion and exclusion criteria tend to select patients who do not resemble patients in actual practice based on age, comorbidities, sex, race/ethnicity, or socioeconomic status. In addition, because sample sizes are usually limited by cost, individual-level trials can rarely address questions about how intervention effects may vary in different subgroups (Armstrong, 2012). Failure to identify this effect, termed treatment heterogeneity, may mean that high-risk subgroups miss the potential benefits of a preventive service if it is found ineffective in the general population. These limitations are not inherent to RCTs; they may also hinder non-randomized studies of interventions. Conversely, many pragmatic or effectiveness trials do enroll patients representative of those in practice.

Modern Trial Designs

Newer designs for RCTs may be useful to overcome specific limitations of individual-level trials. Many excellent books on study design and reviews of modern study methods are available and provide more comprehensive descriptions of the options. Here, the committee discusses selected designs that may be useful in clinical prevention. Examples of modern trial designs include

- **Cluster-randomized trials,** in which the unit of intervention is a group of patients clustered based on an organizing factor such as a clinic, a medical center, or a geographic area. Such designs make it feasible to include large numbers of patients and sometimes do not require individual-level consent.

  Cluster randomization may be especially useful when it would be difficult to provide different interventions to individuals within the same clinical setting. For example, a trial of mailed and telephone intervention to reduce postpartum weight retention among women with gestational diabetes mellitus used a cluster randomized design in order to leverage a centralized system for case management across the 44 medical facilities participating, and to enable consistent workflow within each medical facility.

  Stepped wedge cluster randomized trials are increasingly used to evaluate interventions that involve service delivery in discrete units such as geographical regions, hospitals or clinics. In this design, each unit crosses over from control to intervention in a randomized and sequential fashion (Hemming et al., 2015). This design enables researchers to conduct rigorous evaluation within the constraints sometimes imposed by policy makers when they believe it important that every unit in a study should eventually receive the intervention.
- **Pragmatic RCTs** are designed to test the effectiveness of interventions in real-life clinical practice settings, to maximize applicability and generalizability. They usually have less strict eligibility requirements than individual-level trials and often use cluster randomization. Many focus on outcomes that are measured routinely in the course of usual clinical care. Advantages of pragmatic trials include greater generalizability to diverse populations, ability to enroll larger numbers of patients, and lower cost. For example, a pragmatic randomized trial of one-step versus two-step screening for gestational diabetes was able to study 23,792 women and to study multiple outcomes for both the mothers and infants (Hillier et al., 2021). The trial was pragmatic in that there were few restrictions on interventions subsequent to

screening. It was supported by a National Institutes of Health R01 grant, which is a modest scope for a study of this size

- **Adaptive trial designs** may be useful for situations where an intervention is warranted but where there are multiple possible approaches and the best choice of intervention is initially unclear. In an adaptive trial, the trial protocol includes a planned schedule of assessments and the trial parameters may be modified after each assessment. The parameters that may be modified include the intervention itself, the dosage of a medication, the patient selection criteria, and the sample size. For example, the USPSTF recommends colorectal cancer screening and calls for more research to understand uptake and adherence to individual screening tests, including repeated colonoscopy after 10 years and repeated stool tests annually, as well as research on the accuracy and effectiveness of serum- and urine-based tests ("liquid biopsy" screening) and capsule endoscopy tests, which could enhance adherence. An adaptive trial design might be useful to compare several of these approaches, eliminate less-promising options early in the process, and focus research effort on those with highest potential for benefit.
- **Platform trials** are designed to simultaneously investigate multiple interventions using specialized statistical methods (Berry et al., 2015). This type of trial has been used to study treatments in cancer, infectious diseases, and neurology and is particularly suited to study multiple interventions in heterogeneous populations that need long-term follow-up. Randomization may use adaptive approaches in response to emerging information about the effectiveness of an intervention. Platform trials could be applied to study preventive interventions where simultaneous comparison of three or more approaches in diverse populations is warranted.
- **Effectiveness-implementation hybrid designs** were created to speed the development of evidence useful to implementation while the effectiveness of a service is still being evaluated. "Design" refers to the procedures used to select units or participants for study, assign these to intervention or usual care, and make evaluations before, during, and after study assignment (Landes et al., 2020). Hybrid design denotes that these procedures may have varying degrees of focus on both the effectiveness and implementation of a clinical intervention. The effectiveness-implementation hybrid design is not limited to RCTs. These designs have been used in many studies of behavioral interventions and are discussed in a review by researchers with the Veterans Affairs

Quality Enhancement Research Initiative (Landes et al., 2020). Clinical trials may sometimes be adapted in ways that specifically suit the evaluation of preventive interventions. Examples include trials that help elucidate mechanisms of why interventions have an impact, enable study of the indirect effects of a program or policy, or facilitate collaborations with implementers of preventive services (Alsan and Finkelstein, 2021). In addition, a novel preference-informed complementary trial design may help trials include patients with strong preferences who might decline to enroll in a traditionally designed trial (Ali et al., 2021).

OBSERVATIONAL STUDY DESIGNS

Observational study designs for comparative effectiveness compare a group that has been exposed to a condition or intervention (e.g., screening or treatment) with a comparison group that has not. Historically, observational studies have been plagued with biases, also referred to as confounding. These include selection bias (when the intervention and comparison groups differ in characteristics associated with the outcome of interest) and performance bias (when delivery of an intervention is associated with generally higher levels of quality of care by the health care unit) (Armstrong, 2012).

Cohort study designs are prone to problems that threaten their internal validity, including secular trend and regression to the mean. Multivariable analysis is perhaps the oldest and best-established method of adjusting for confounders that have been measured. However, specific well-known cases have underscored the limitations of cohort study designs, even when they include untreated comparison groups and multivariable analysis is applied. For example, multiple observational studies prior to the late 1990s indicated that the use of postmenopausal hormone replacement therapy was associated with substantial reduction in coronary heart disease risk (Humphrey et al., 2002). Subsequently, a large RCT of postmenopausal hormone replacement therapy (HRT) found no benefit in cardiovascular heart disease (CHD) risk (Rossouw et al., 2002). This apparent contradiction stemmed in part from many of the observational studies not having collected data on socioeconomic status, which was a key confounder of the relationship between HRT use and CHD risk.

It should be noted that in research intended to reduce health disparities for underrepresented individuals, the control group (both in RCTs and observational designs) should be selected to be as similar as possible to the intervention group. Recent articles recommend standards for reporting on race and ethnicity (Flanagin et al., 2021) and for research and publication on racial health inequities (Boyd et al., 2020).

In recent years, newer study designs and analytic methods have offered more robust approaches for causal inference, the process of inferring that an action or event affects an outcome of interest (Rothman and Greenland, 2005). Modern analytic methods include

- **Propensity score methods,** which are analytic approaches used in observational studies to balance the intervention and comparison groups on observed pre-intervention characteristics. For each study subject, the researcher generates a propensity score that reflects the individual's likelihood of receiving the intervention based on their characteristics. Propensity scores are discussed in many review articles (Glynn et al., 2006; Luo et al., 2010; Stürmer et al., 2014) and can be used in several different ways, including adjusting the multivariable regression analysis or matching subjects who received the intervention with appropriate comparison subjects. The use of propensity scores may be especially useful in studies evaluating real-world effectiveness after a preventive service has been recommended.
- **Instrumental variable analysis,** which uses a variable to separate study subjects into two groups, one of which is more likely to have received an intervention than another (Martens et al., 2006). It is typically used retrospectively. The use of the variable, termed the instrumental variable, attempts to mimic random assignment to the intervention vs. the control group. The requirement is that the instrumental variable be associated with the exposure or intervention of interest, but not with the outcome. One advantage of instrumental variable design is that, in theory, it controls for unmeasured confounders. One disadvantage of this approach that there are few situations where an ideal instrumental variable exists, because many prospective instrumental variables are associated with the outcome to some extent.

  For example, if a behavioral intervention to prevent illicit drug use in adolescents were made available only to patients making clinic visits on Mondays, Wednesdays, and Fridays, the day of the week each clinic visit was made might be usable as an instrumental variable in an observational study, provided it were not associated with the outcomes of interest.

Quasi-experimental designs can be used to enhance the robustness of non-randomized studies of interventions (Harris et al., 2006). Examples include

- **Difference-in-difference design** (nonrandomized trial with comparison group). In this design, outcomes are initially measured at a baseline time point in two similar groups. Then, one group receives the intervention while the comparison group does not. Subsequently, outcomes are measured again, usually at the same time point for each group. This design can be used prospectively (in advance of data collection) or retrospectively (on existing data). It mitigates secular trend and regression to the mean, both of which are inherent flaws in study designs that involve observing only the group that receives an intervention.

  This design can be useful when it is impossible to assign multiple groups at random to intervention or control. For example, if one health care system initiated a program that focused on enhancing colorectal cancer screening through annual stool testing, its outcomes before and after the program began could be compared with a similar system without such a program.
- **Interrupted time-series design** is often used to study changes in health care policy, such as changes in guidelines, laws, or financing mechanisms. In these situations, it is generally impossible to randomize, and the policy change usually occurs at a single point in time. If the policy change has an effect on an outcome, researchers observing the rate of the outcome over time will see a sudden change in the slope of the curve at the time of the policy change. This design is best used to study policy changes that take effect all at once rather than gradually, and can only be used when data are available from enough time points before and after the policy change. For example, if a health care financing policy changed to provide access to a preventive service that was previously unavailable to a group of patients, and if uptake of the preventive service were brisk, this design could be used to study the resulting changes in outcomes.

PREDICTIVE ANALYTICS

Most of the recent USPSTF statements the committee reviewed called for predictive analytics—risk prediction studies using tests, questionnaires, or clinical characteristics to identify patients at high risk for a condition. Research needs involving predictive analytics can be categorized as studying physical screening tests (e.g., laboratory, imaging, colonoscopy), clinical examination findings (e.g., visual examination for skin cancer), patient-reported factors on questionnaires, other clinical characteristics, or combinations of these.

A rich body of literature exists on methods for evaluating test performance and setting test cutoffs. Some common methods and issues to consider include the need for prediction models to have adequate discrimination and calibration (Alba et al., 2017), and the use of receiver operating characteristic curves to identify potential test cutoff points (Poldrack et al., 2020).

The importance of predictive analytics in clinical prevention research is likely to increase in the foreseeable future due to scientific advances that create the opportunity for precision medicine and precision public health. Genomics, proteomics, and metabolomics are among the many biological fields that could provide new tools for clinical prevention by developing tests to identify patient groups at high risk of future disease. Advances in artificial intelligence have made it possible to analyze images and text and to generate computer-based predictive algorithms using myriad variables available in electronic health records. Patient monitoring technology that gathers highly detailed data, such as wearable patches for heart rhythm monitoring in atrial fibrillation, is also increasing. These trends are likely to increase the needs for predictive analytics, and for modeling studies that combine predictive analytic methods with other methods to give a comprehensive overview of the projected benefits and harms of a preventive service.

One issue that seems likely to warrant increasing attention by researchers and guideline committees is the need to conduct studies that evaluate the net incremental value of a test or prediction model (i.e., its additional value relative to existing methods of identifying patients as high risk). For example, the USPSTF statement on risk assessment of cardiovascular disease using nontraditional risk factors (including the ankle-brachial index, high-sensitivity C-reactive protein, and coronary artery calcification score) noted that studies assessing these factors in isolation are of limited value. Instead, the statement called for studies comparing traditional risk assessment with traditional risk assessment plus one or more of the newer factors, so that the incremental benefits and harms of the newer factors can be more clearly delineated. Likewise, in studies of computer-based risk prediction models, Shah et al. (2019) have called for considering the net incremental value of taking plausible actions when selecting the best model, rather than simply relying on statistical measures.

MODELING

Modeling refers to the use of tables or computer-based simulations to make projections about outcomes under varying scenarios. Models range from simple calculations presented in outcomes tables to more formal decision models. The USPSTF uses modeling to inform recommendations when there is direct evidence of the benefit of a preventive service on health outcomes, or when there is evidence for each of the linkages in an analytic framework. The USPSTF Procedure Manual notes that candidates for modeling are generally A, B, and some C recommendations, and notes that decision modeling is primarily warranted when there are outstanding clinical questions about how best to target a clinical preventive service at the individual and program level, and it is unlikely that the systematic review can confidently determine the magnitude of net benefit, particularly for subpopulations of interest (USPSTF, 2021). Thus, the USPSTF currently uses modeling in a highly focused way, to further inform the applications of letter grade recommendations to subpopulations. It would not use modeling to overturn an "insufficient evidence" statement.

Modeling has potentially important uses in research on preventive services beyond its current role in the USPSTF process. For example, a research sponsor with finite funding may wish to compare the value of investing in research on one preventive services topic compared with another, or within a given topic, compare the value of investing in studies to address one key question compared with another. Decision models could be used to project the potential findings of the proposed studies, their effects on preventive services recommendations, and the downstream effects on health outcomes. Multi-criteria decision analysis, a type of decision modeling that takes into account multiple factors of interest, could be used along with the prioritization criteria in the taxonomy presented in this report. Such models could help sponsors compare the projected costs, benefits, and perceived value of alternative investments in research.

Modeling could also be used to inform some of the challenging decisions among competing priorities in preventive care that clinicians and policy makers make in real-world practice. For example, the number of preventive services recommended during an average visit may exceed the amount of time a clinician has available to address them. In addition, many patients have comorbidities that set up competing priorities with the impetus to deliver preventive care. To present realistic projections of the impact of preventive services in actual practice, it would be helpful for models to not assume 100 percent adherence to an intervention and to account for the fact that harms and benefits data from randomized trials may need to be adjusted to reflect real-world outcomes.

Decision models are inherently imperfect and usually rely on base case assumptions about which uncertainty exists. Sensitivity analysis is important in all modeling, to understand how results may change when assumptions are varied over plausible ranges. With the appropriate caveats in mind, modeling can be helpful to elucidate the tradeoffs among costs, benefits, and harms of alternative options, to support decision making by policy makers, operational leaders of programs that deliver preventive care, and individual clinicians and patients.

RESEARCH ON GROUP DECISION PROCESSES

The USPSTF is one of many groups that develop recommendations on preventive services, and its methods are highly evidence-based and structured compared with most others. Even with its highly evolved approaches, the task force likely still has room for additional refinement in the processes used to arrive at decisions as a group. These processes could be applied, for example, to help the task force determine priorities among evidence gaps identified via the use of the taxonomy.

One example of structured group communication and decision-making processes is the Delphi method, which uses iterative questionnaires and statistical feedback to the group to develop a consensus. Other quantitative methods of group decision making include voting, weighting, ranking, scoring, and grading (Madhavan et al., 2017). Some methods, including multi-criteria decision analysis and analytic hierarchy process, enable the user to assign weights to different criteria that describe the options; this can be used for individual or group decision-making (Phelps and Madhavan, 2017). These methods are often poorly understood and deserve to be subjected to more practical research.

The USPSTF uses several types of processes where methods for group decision-making could be further tested and refined, including the selection of topics to review, the decision about a recommendation on a given topic once the evidence is reviewed, and in the future, the prioritization among evidence gaps that should be filled for a given topic. Learning more about how to best apply such methods in developing recommendations on preventive services and associated research would enhance the robustness of decisions and optimize their downstream impact.

REFERENCES

Alba, A. C., T. Agoritsas, M. Walsh, S. Hanna, A. Iorio, P. J. Devereaux, T. McGinn, and G. Guyatt. 2017. Discrimination and calibration of clinical prediction models: Users' guides to the medical literature. *JAMA* 318(14):1377–1384.

Ali, S., G. Hopkin, N. Poonai, L. Richer, M. Yaskina, A. Heath, T. P. Klassen, C. McCabe, KidsCAN PERC Innovative Pediatric Clinical Trials No OUCH Study Group, and KidsCAN PERC Innovative Pediatric Clinical Trials Methods Core. 2021. Correction to: A novel preference-informed complementary trial (PICT) design for clinical trial research influenced by strong patient preferences. *Trials* 22(1):353.

Alsan, M. and A. N. Finkelstein. 2021. Beyond causality: Additional benefits of randomized controlled trials for improving health care delivery. *The Milbank Quarterly*.

Armstrong, K. 2012. Methods in comparative effectiveness research. *Journal of Clinical Oncology* 30(34):4208–4214.

Berry, S. M., J. T. Connor, and R. J. Lewis. 2015. The platform trial: An efficient strategy for evaluating multiple treatments. *JAMA* 313(16):1619–1620.

Boyd, R. W., E. G. Lindo, L. D. Weeks, and M. R. McLemore. 2020. On racism: A new standard for publishing on racial health inequities. *Health Affairs Blog*, July 2, 2020. https://www.healthaffairs.org/do/10.1377/hblog20200630.939347/full (accessed November 1, 2021).

Flanagin, A., T. Frey, S. L. Christiansen, and AMA Manual of Style Committee. 2021. Updated guidance on the reporting of race and ethnicity in medical and science journals. *JAMA* 326(7):621–627.

Glynn, R. J., S. Schneeweiss, and T. Stürmer. 2006. Indications for propensity scores and review of their use in pharmacoepidemiology. *Basic & Clinical Pharmacology & Toxicology* 98(3):253–259.

Guyatt, G., A. D. Oxman, E. A. Akl, R. Kunz, G. Vist, J. Brozek, S. Norris, Y. Falck-Ytter, P. Glasziou, H. DeBeer, R. Jaeschke, D. Rind, J. Meerpohl, P. Dahm, and H. J. Schünemann. 2011. GRADE guidelines: 1. Introduction—GRADE evidence profiles and summary of findings tables. *Journal of Clinical Epidemiology* 64(4):383–394.

Harris, A. D., J. C. McGregor, E. N. Perencevich, J. P. Furuno, J. Zhu, D. E. Peterson, and J. Finkelstein. 2006. The use and interpretation of quasi-experimental studies in medical informatics. *Journal of the American Medical Informatics Association* 13(1):16–23.

Hemming, K., T. P. Haines, P. J. Chilton, A. J. Girling, and R. J. Lilford. 2015. The stepped wedge cluster randomised trial: Rationale, design, analysis, and reporting. *BMJ* 350:h391.

Hillier, T. A., K. L. Pedula, K. K. Ogasawara, K. K. Vesco, C. E. S. Oshiro, S. L. Lubarsky, and J. Van Marter. 2021. A pragmatic, randomized clinical trial of gestational diabetes screening. *New England Journal of Medicine* 384(10):895–904.

Humphrey, L. L., B. K. S. Chan, and H. C. Sox, Jr. 2002. Postmenopausal hormone replacement therapy and the primary prevention of cardiovascular disease. *Annals of Internal Medicine* 137(4):273–284.

Landes, S. J., S. A. McBain, and G. M. Curran. 2020. Reprint of: An introduction to effectiveness-implementation hybrid designs. *Psychiatry Research* 283(16):112630.

Luo, Z., J. C. Gardiner, and C. J. Bradley. 2010. Applying propensity score methods in medical research: Pitfalls and prospects. *Medical Care Research and Review* 67(5):528–554.

Madhavan, G., C. Phelps, and R. Rappuoli. 2017. Compare voting systems to improve them. *Nature* 541(7636):151–153.

Martens, E. P., W. R. Pestman, A. d. Boer, S. V. Belitser, and O. H. Klungel. 2006. Instrumental variables: Application and limitations. *Epidemiology* 17(3):260–267.

Phelps, C. E., and G. Madhavan. 2017. Using multicriteria approaches to assess the value of health care. *Value Health* 20(2):251–255.

Poldrack, R. A., G. Huckins, and G. Varoquaux. 2020. Establishment of best practices for evidence for prediction: A review. *JAMA Psychiatry* 77(5):534–540.

Rossouw, J. E., G. L. Anderson, R. L. Prentice, A. Z. LaCroix, C. Kooperberg, M. L. Stefanick, R. D. Jackson, S. A. A. Beresford, B. V. Howard, K. C. Johnson, J. M. Kotchen, J. Ockene, and Writing Group for the Women's Health Initiative Investigators. 2002. Risks and benefits of estrogen plus progestin in healthy postmenopausal women: Principal results from the women's health initiative randomized controlled trial. *JAMA* 288(3):321–333.

Rothman, K. J., and S. Greenland. 2005. Causation and causal inference in epidemiology. *American Journal of Public Health* 95:S144–S150.

Schünemann, H. J., C. Cuello, E. A. Akl, R. A. Mustafa, J. J. Meerpohl, K. Thayer, R. L. Morgan, G. Gartlehner, R. Kunz, S. V. Katikireddi, J. Sterne, J. P. Higgins, G. Guyatt, and G. W. Group. 2019. Grade guidelines: 18. How ROBINS-I and other tools to assess risk of bias in nonrandomized studies should be used to rate the certainty of a body of evidence. *Journal of Clinical Epidemiology* 111:105–114.

Shah, N. H., A. Milstein, and S. C. Bagley. 2019. Making machine learning models clinically useful. *JAMA* 322(14):1351–1352.

Sterne, J. A., M. A. Hernán, B. C. Reeves, J. Savović, N. D. Berkman, M. Viswanathan, D. Henry, D. G. Altman, M. T. Ansari, I. B. I., J. R. Carpenter, A. W. Chan, R. Churchill, J. J. Deeks, A. Hróbjartsson, J. Kirkham, P. J. P., Y. K. Loke, T. D. Pigott, C. R. Ramsay, D. Regidor, H. R. Rothstein, L. Sandhu, P. L. Santaguida, H. J. Schünemann, B. Shea, I. Shrier, P. Tugwell, L. Turner, J. C. Valentine, H. Waddington, E. Waters, G. A. Wells, P. F. Whiting, and J. P. Higgins. 2016. ROBINS-I: A tool for assessing risk of bias in non-randomised studies of interventions. *BMJ* 355:i4919.

Stürmer, T., R. Wyss, R. J. Glynn, and M. A. Brookhart. 2014. Propensity scores for confounder adjustment when assessing the effects of medical interventions using nonexperimental study designs. *Journal of Internal Medicine* 275(6):570–580.

USPSTF (U.S. Preventive Services Task Force). 2021. *U.S. Preventive Services Task Force procedure manual.* https://www.uspreventiveservicestaskforce.org/uspstf/about-uspstf/methods-and-processes/procedure-manual (accessed August 30, 2021).

C

Public Meeting Agendas

FIRST PUBLIC MEETING
December 15, 2020
Videoconference via Zoom

11:00 AM **Welcome and Introductions**
- Tracy Lieu, M.D., M.P.H., *Committee Chair; Director,* Kaiser Permanente Northern California Division of Research

11:10 AM **AHRQ Perspective on the Statement of Task**
- Arlene Bierman, M.D., M.S., *Director,* Center for Evidence and Practice Improvement, AHRQ

11:20 AM **NIH Perspective on the Statement of Task**
- David Murray, Ph.D., *Associate Director for Prevention and Director,* Office of Disease Prevention, NIH

11:30 AM **Discussion**

12:00 PM **The Role of the USPSTF in Identifying Evidence Gaps**
- Amanda Borsky, Dr.P.H., M.P.P., *Program Manager,* U.S. Preventive Services Task Force Program, AHRQ

- Carol M. Mangione, M.D., M.S.P.H., FACP, *Chief*, Division of General Medicine and Health Services Research; *Barbara A. Levey & Gerald S. Levey Professor of Medicine and Public Health*, UCLA; *USPSTF Vice-Chair*

12:25 PM **The Role of NIH in Addressing Evidence Gaps**
- Carrie Klabunde, Ph.D., *Senior Advisor for Disease Prevention*, Office of Disease Prevention, NIH

12:40 PM **Discussion**

1:00 PM **Adjourn**

SECOND PUBLIC MEETING
March 4, 2021
Videoconference via Zoom

11:00 AM **Welcome and Introductions**
- Tracy Lieu, M.D., M.P.H., *Committee Chair; Director*, Kaiser Permanente Northern California Division of Research

11:10 AM **Pathways to Addressing Evidence Gaps**
- Chyke A. Doubeni, M.D., M.P.H., *Member*, USPSTF; *Director*, Mayo Clinic Center for Health Equity and Community Engagement Research
- Paul Doria-Rose, Ph.D., D.V.M., *Chief*, Healthcare Assessment Research Branch, Health Delivery Research Program, Division of Cancer Control and Population Sciences, NCI
- Doug Corley, M.D., Ph.D., *Lead Investigator*, NCI PROSPR Consortium; *Research Scientist*, Kaiser Permanente Northern California Division of Research

11:40 AM **Moderated Discussion**

12:35 PM **Break**

12:40 PM **Taxonomy: Categorizing Evidence Gaps in Order to Address Them**
- Alex H. Krist, M.D., M.P.H., *Chair*, USPSTF; *Professor of Family Medicine and Population Health*, Virginia Commonwealth University

- Karen A. Robinson, Ph.D., M.Sc., *Director*, Evidence-Based Practice Center, Johns Hopkins University
- Susan J. Curry, Ph.D., *Senior Advisor for Preventive Services*, NIH; *Dean Emerita and Distinguished Professor of Health Management and Policy*, University of Iowa

1:10 PM **Moderated Discussion**

2:00 PM **Adjourn**

THIRD PUBLIC MEETING
March 16, 2021
Videoconference via Zoom

11:00 AM **Welcome and Introductions**

- Tracy Lieu, M.D., M.P.H., *Committee Chair; Director,* Kaiser Permanente Northern California Division of Research

11:10 AM **Perspectives on Addressing Evidence Gaps: The CDC Community Guide**

- Amy Lansky, Ph.D., M.P.H., *Director*, CDC Community Guide

11:20 AM **Perspectives on Addressing Evidence Gaps: Funders**

- Michael S. Lauer, M.D., *Deputy Director for Extramural Research*, NIH
- Harold (Hal) Sox, M.D., *Director*, Peer Review, PCORI
- David Atkins, M.D., M.P.H., *Director of Health Services Research & Development*, VA

11:50 AM **Moderated Discussion**

12:10 PM **Break**

12:15 PM **Case Example: Autism Screening "I" Statement Impact on the Research Community**

- Michael Silverstein, M.D., M.P.H., *Member*, USPSTF; *Professor of Pediatrics, Director of the Division of General Academic Pediatrics,* and *Vice Chair of Research for the Department of Pediatrics,* Boston University School of Medicine

- Ann E. Wagner, Ph.D., *Department of Health and Human Services National Autism Coordinator*, Office of NIMH Director, NIMH, NIH
- Sarabeth Broder-Fingert, M.D., M.P.H., *Associate Professor of Pediatrics*, Boston University School of Medicine; *Co-Director*, Innovation in Autism Disparities, Inclusion, Outreach, and Transition Services Lab, Boston University

12:30 PM **Moderated Discussion**

1:05 PM **Reflections on a Taxonomy of Evidence Gaps and Research to Close Them**

- Ned Calonge, M.D., M.P.H., *President and Chief Executive Officer*, Colorado Trust; *Associate Professor of Family Medicine*, Colorado School of Medicine, and *Associate Professor of Epidemiology*, Colorado School of Public Health, University of Colorado Denver
- Alan I. Leshner, Ph.D., *Chief Executive Officer Emeritus*, AAAS, and *Executive Publisher*, *Science* Magazine; *Former Director*, NIDA; *Former Deputy Director and Acting Director*, NIMH

2:00 PM **Adjourn**

FOURTH PUBLIC MEETING
June 24, 2021
Videoconference via Zoom

11:30 AM **Welcome**

- Tracy Lieu, M.D., M.P.H., *Committee Chair*; *Director*, Kaiser Permanente Northern California Division of Research

11:35 AM **NIH Stories of Success in Disease Prevention: Informing National Recommendations about Clinical Preventive Services**

- Carrie Klabunde, Ph.D., *Senior Advisor for Disease Prevention*, Office of Disease Prevention, NIH

12:15 PM **Adjourn**

D

Committee Member and Staff Biographies

COMMITTEE MEMBERS

Tracy A. Lieu, M.D., M.P.H., is the director of the Division of Research for Kaiser Permanente Northern California. She leads a group of 600 people who conduct studies in clinical effectiveness, delivery science, and epidemiology to enhance the health of Kaiser Permanente members and society at large. Dr. Lieu is a practicing pediatrician who has led nationally recognized work in vaccine safety and policy and childhood asthma. Previously, Dr. Lieu was a professor and the founding director of the Center for Child Health Care Studies in the Department of Population Medicine at Harvard Pilgrim Health Care Institute and Harvard Medical School. Her national roles have included membership on the U.S. Preventive Services Task Force and the Advisory Committee on Immunization Practices and the chair of the Health Services Organization and Delivery study section of the National Institutes of Health. She has served on three previous National Academies consensus study committees. Dr. Lieu has an M.D. from the University of California, San Francisco, and an M.P.H. from the University of California, Berkeley. She is an elected member of the National Academy of Medicine.

Cathy J. Bradley, Ph.D., M.P.A., is a professor and the associate dean for research at the Colorado School of Public Health and the deputy director of the University of Colorado Cancer Center. She holds the Bunn Chair in Cancer Research. Prior to joining the University of Colorado, she was the founding chair of the Department of Healthcare Policy and Research and the associate director of cancer prevention and control at the Virginia Commonwealth University School of Medicine. Dr. Bradley is an internationally recognized expert in health services research and health economics. Her expertise is in labor market outcomes of cancer survivors, health policy, and health disparities. Dr. Bradley is on the editorial board of the *Journal of Cancer Survivorship*. She has previously served on a National Academies consensus study committee and currently serves on the National Cancer Policy Forum. Dr. Bradley has a Ph.D. and an M.P.A. from the University of North Carolina at Chapel Hill.

Theodore G. Ganiats, M.D., is a professor emeritus in family medicine and public health at the University of California, San Diego (UCSD). Dr. Ganiats is a member of many professional associations, including the Society for Medical Decision Making, AcademyHealth, the American Public Health Association, and the International Society for Quality of Life Research. He was the founder and the first executive director of the UCSD Health Services Research Center. While representing the American Academy of Family Physicians, Dr. Ganiats reviewed dozens of reports for the U.S. Preventive Services Task Force. He has served as a member or the chair of more than 50 national guideline, quality, and performance panels spanning multiple disciplines. He served as the director of the National Center for Excellence in Primary Care Research at the Agency for Healthcare Research and Quality. He has previously served on two National Academies consensus study committees. Dr. Ganiats has an M.D. from UCSD. He is an elected member of the National Academy of Medicine.

Keng-Yen Huang, Ph.D., M.P.H., M.A., is an associate professor of population health and child and adolescent psychiatry at the New York University Grossman School of Medicine. Dr. Huang is a co-investigator of the African Center for Collaborative Child Mental Health Implementation Research, which aims to build capacity for evidence-based child behavioral health policy and implementation research in Uganda, Ghana, and Kenya. In addition, she serves as the principal investigator and co-investigator on numerous child development and mental health implementation research projects in international contexts. Dr. Huang is a prevention and translational researcher with strong expertise across multiple disciplines, including epidemiology, behavioral health, pediatric health and development, health disparities, global public health, implementation and dissemination science, and health policy and management. Her current research efforts focus on child mental and behavioral health implementation and epidemiological research in primary care and in community service contexts both in low- and middle-income countries and in the

United States. Dr. Huang has a Ph.D. and an M.A. from the University of Maryland, Baltimore, and an M.P.H. from New York University.

Preeti Gokal Kochar, Ph.D., is a technical information specialist at the National Library of Medicine (NLM) at the National Institutes of Health. At NLM, Dr. Kochar analyzes biomedical journal articles and assigns the relevant Medical Subject Headings (MeSH). She previously created and led a team that made a prototype of an app that uses MeSH taxonomy to create a visualization to search PubMed. Dr. Kochar works on projects involving data science, and her goal is to use data science to turn biomedical information into knowledge. Currently, she is leading a team to programmatically identify new concepts in PubMed/MEDLINE citations as part of NLM's Indexing Automation effort. Her areas of expertise include controlled vocabularies, information retrieval, literature-based discovery, genetics, molecular biology, and biochemistry. Dr. Kochar has a Ph.D. from the University of South Carolina.

Ann E. Kurth, Ph.D., C.N.M., M.P.H., M.S.N., is the dean and the Linda Koch Lorimer Professor at the Yale University School of Nursing and a professor of epidemiology at the Yale School of Public Health. As an epidemiologist and clinically trained nurse-midwife, Dr. Kurth's research focuses on HIV/reproductive health and global health system strengthening, particularly in the context of climate change. Dr. Kurth has published more than 200 peer-reviewed articles, book chapters, and scholarly monographs and has presented at hundreds of scientific conferences and invited talks. She has received awards for her science and leadership including the Friends of the National Institute of Nursing Research Award and the International Nurse Researcher Hall of Fame award from Sigma Theta Tau International, the global nursing honor society. Dr. Kurth is a former member of the U.S. Preventive Services Task Force, a current member of the New York Academy of Medicine and the CT Academy of Science and Engineering, and a fellow of the American Academy of Nursing. She has previously served on two National Academies consensus study committees and currently chairs the Board on Global Health. Dr. Kurth has a Ph.D. from the University of Washington; an M.S.N., R.N., and C.S.N. from Yale University in Connecticut; and an M.P.H. from Columbia University in New York. She is an elected member of the National Academy of Medicine.

Tianjing Li, M.D., Ph.D., M.H.S., is an associate professor in the Department of Ophthalmology at the University of Colorado (CU) Anschutz Medical Campus with a secondary appointment in the Department of Epidemiology at the CU School of Public Health. Prior to her roles at CU,

Dr. Li worked as an associate professor in the Department of Epidemiology at the Johns Hopkins Bloomberg School of Public Health (JHBSPH). The primary focus of Dr. Li's research is to develop, evaluate, and disseminate efficient methods for comparing health care interventions and to provide trustworthy evidence for decision making. Dr. Li holds leadership roles within Cochrane, including serving as the associate director for Cochrane United States from 2012 to 2018, a coordinating editor for *Cochrane Eyes and Vision* since 2018, a co-convener for the Cochrane Comparing Multiple Interventions Methods Group since 2011, and a member of the Cochrane Methods Executive Committee since 2019. Dr. Li was the 2019 recipient of Cochrane's Anne Anderson Award, which recognized her cumulative accomplishment, originality, and independence of thought, leadership, and inspiration for women within Cochrane. Dr. Li is the president elect of the Society for Research Synthesis Methodology. She serves as the Society's secretary and received its inaugural Early Career Award in 2016. Dr. Li has previously served on a National Academies consensus study committee. She has an M.D. from Sichuan University in China, and a Ph.D. and an M.H.S. from JHBSPH.

K. M. Venkat Narayan, M.D., M.Sc., M.B.A., is the director of the Emory Global Diabetes Research Center, a professor of global health and epidemiology at the Emory Rollins School of Public Health, and a professor of medicine at the Emory University School of Medicine. Dr. Narayan studies diabetes and noncommunicable disease pathophysiology, epidemiology, control, prevention, and policy. He has been involved in scientific leadership of several major national and international multi-center epidemiological studies, public health surveillance, translation research, intervention studies, economic models, and health policy. Dr. Narayan has previously served on two National Academies consensus study committees. He has an M.D. from St. John's Medical College in India, an M.Sc. from the University of Edinburgh, and an M.B.A from Herriot Watt University in Scotland. Dr. Narayan is an elected member of the National Academy of Medicine.

Wanda K. Nicholson, M.D., M.P.H., M.B.A., is the chair of the American College of Obstetricians and Gynecologists' Working Group on Diversity, Equity, and Inclusive Excellence and serves on the Board of Directors for the American Board of Obstetrics and Gynecology. She is a practicing obstetrician-gynecologist in North Carolina and a researcher in population health and health equity, population improvement, and access to care for rural populations. Her research focus centers on social determinants of health and management of diabetes and cardiovascular disease. Dr. Nicholson works to develop research performance measures for value-based care and better health outcomes. She is an associate editor for the *American Journal of Obstetrics and Gynecology* and a former member of the U.S. Preventive Services Task Force. Dr. Nicholson has an M.D. from the University of North Carolina at Chapel Hill, an M.P.H. from the University of California, Berkeley, and an M.B.A. from Johns Hopkins University in Maryland.

Elizabeth O. Ofili, M.D., M.P.H., FACC, is a professor of medicine at the Morehouse School of Medicine and the chief medical officer of the Morehouse Choice Accountable Care Organization in Georgia. Dr. Ofili is a national and internationally recognized clinician scientist with particular focus on cardiovascular disparities and women's health. As the president of the Association of Black Cardiologists, she led the initiative to implement the landmark African American Heart Failure Trial, whose findings led to a change in practice guidelines for the treatment of heart failure in African Americans. She has previously served on a National Academies consensus study committee and currently serves on the Roundtable on the Black Men and Black Women in Science, Engineering, and Medicine. Dr. Ofili has an M.D. from Ahmadu Bello University in Nigeria and an M.P.H. from Johns Hopkins University in Maryland. She is an elected member of the National Academy of Medicine.

Nicolaas P. Pronk, Ph.D., M.A., is the president of HealthPartners Institute and the chief science officer at HealthPartners in Minnesota. He serves as the co-chair of the U.S. Secretary of Health and Human Services' Advisory Committee on National Health Promotion and Disease Prevention Objectives for 2030. In addition, he holds a faculty appointment as an adjunct professor of social and behavioral sciences at the Harvard T.H. Chan School of Public Health in Massachusetts and an affiliate full professor of health policy and management at the University of Minnesota School of Public Health. Dr. Pronk's work is focused on connecting evidence of effectiveness with practical applications of programs, practices, policies, and systems that measurably improve population health and well-being. He is a former member of the Community Preventive Services Task Force and the Defense Health Board. He has previously served on four National Academies consensus study committees and currently chairs the Roundtable on Obesity Solutions. Dr. Pronk has a Ph.D. from Texas A&M University College Station and an M.A. from Kearney State College in Nebraska.

Robert B. Wallace, M.D., M.Sc., is the Irene Ensminger Stecher Emeritus Professor of Epidemiology and Internal Medicine at the University of Iowa College of Public Health. He is currently involved in several active research projects funded by the National Institutes of Health. He has conducted many population health studies and clinical trials focusing on the prevention and control of chronic illnesses and other disabling conditions of older persons. Dr. Wallace was a member of the U.S. Preventive Services Task Force and the National Advisory Council on Aging of the National Institute on Aging and is a fellow of the American College of Preventive Medicine. He received the National Academy of Medicine's Walsh McDermott Medal in recognition for his distinguished service, having participated in more than 20 National Academies consensus study committees. Dr. Wallace has an M.D. from Northwestern University in Illinois and an M.Sc. from State University of New York at Buffalo. He is an elected member of the National Academy of Medicine.

STAFF

Kathleen R. Stratton, Ph.D., serves as the study director for the Committee on Addressing Evidence Gaps in Clinical Prevention Recommendations. Dr. Stratton began her career at the National Academies of Sciences, Engineering, and Medicine in 1990 in the Institute of Medicine (IOM). She has spent most of her time with the Board on Population Health and Public Health Practice. She has staffed committees addressing vaccine safety and development, pandemic preparedness, environmental and occupational health, drug safety, and tobacco control. Dr. Stratton received the IOM Cecil Research Award for sustained contributions to vaccine safety and was made a staff Scholar in 2005. After 2 years at The Pew Charitable Trusts working on Food and Drug Administration reform, she returned to the National Academies in fall 2013. Dr. Stratton is currently involved in a workshop on sponsor influence on health research. She is also directing one study related to evaluating Substance Abuse and Mental Health Services Administration–funded programs under the Comprehensive Addiction and Recovery Act in addition to this one on addressing research gaps in clinical prevention recommendations. Dr. Stratton received a B.A. in natural sciences from Johns Hopkins University and a Ph.D. in pharmacology and toxicology at the University of Maryland, Baltimore. She conducted postdoctoral research in the Department of Neuroscience at the Johns Hopkins University School of Medicine.

Alexis Wojtowicz is an associate program officer who has supported the National Academies of Sciences, Engineering, and Medicine's Board on Population Health and Public Health Practice since 2016. She has also supported the Roundtable on Health Literacy, an action collaborative on preventing firearm violence, and consensus studies about Medicare payment and the public health effects of e-cigarettes. Before joining the National Academies, Wojtowicz conducted recruitment and intake at a culinary job training program in Washington, DC, and prior to that, coordinated an AmeriCorps VISTA program that placed Summer Associate members at anti-hunger nonprofit organizations across the United States. Wojtowicz has a B.A. in art history from the University of Maryland and is currently pursuing an M.P.H. at the Johns Hopkins Bloomberg School of Public Health, where she is a Bloomberg American Health Initiative Fellow.

Ayshia Coletrane recently joined the National Academies of Sciences, Engineering, and Medicine's Board on Population Health and Public Health Practice as a senior program assistant in 2020. She supports the Roundtable on Population Health Improvement and the consensus study addressing evidence gaps in clinical prevention recommendations. Prior to joining the National Academies, Coletrane taught English as a Fulbright Scholar in Spain. She also conducted research for a study examining the social determinants of health among the Washington, DC, Medicaid population at The George Washington (GW) University Milken Institute School of Public Health, and later coordinated a medical student clerkship under the GW Medical Faculty Associates' Department of Emergency Medicine. Coletrane has a B.S. in health: science, society & policy, and a B.A. in biology from Brandeis University, and is currently pursuing an M.H.A. at The GW Milken Institute School of Public Health.

Rose Marie Martinez, Sc.D., is the senior director of the National Academies' Board on Population Health and Public Health Practice. The board has a vibrant portfolio of studies that address high profile and pressing issues that affect population health. It addresses the science base for population health and public health interventions and examines the capacity of the health system, particularly the public health infrastructure, to support disease prevention and health promotion activities, including educating and supplying the health professionals necessary for carrying them out. The board has examined such topics as the safety of childhood vaccines and other drugs; systems for evaluating and ensuring drug safety after marketing; pandemic influenza planning; the health effects of cannabis and cannabinoids; the health effects of environmental exposures; the integration of medical care and public health; women's health services; health disparities; health literacy; tobacco control strategies; and chronic disease prevention. Before joining the National Academies, Dr. Martinez was a senior health researcher at Mathematica Policy Research, where she conducted research on the impact of health system change on the public health infrastructure, access to care for low-income populations, managed care, and the health care workforce. Dr. Martinez is a former assistant director for health financing and policy with the U.S. General Accounting Office, where she directed evaluations and policy analysis in the area of national and public health issues. Her experience also includes 6 years directing research studies for the Regional Health Ministry of Madrid, Spain. Dr. Martinez is a member of the Council on Education for Public Health, the accreditation body for schools of public health and public health programs. Dr. Martinez received her Sc.D. from the Johns Hopkins University School of Hygiene and Public Health.

E

U.S. Preventive Services Task Force's Reports to Congress[1]

This appendix presents the research gaps and priorities identified by each of the U.S. Preventive Services Task Force's (USPSTF's) annual reports to Congress.

"TENTH ANNUAL REPORT TO CONGRESS ON HIGH-PRIORITY EVIDENCE GAPS FOR CLINICAL PREVENTIVE SERVICES" (2020)

- Child and adolescent health and health inequities related to:
  - Mental and behavioral health
    - Screening for depression in children and adolescents
    - Screening for suicide risk in adolescents, adults, and older adults
  - Substance use
    - Primary care interventions for prevention and cessation of tobacco use in children and adolescents
    - Primary care-based interventions for illicit drug use in children, adolescents, and young adults
    - Screening for unhealthy drug use in adolescents
  - Obesity
    - Screening for obesity in children and adolescents

[1] Adapted from https://www.uspreventiveservicestaskforce.org/uspstf/about-uspstf/reports-congress (accessed July 30, 2021).

"NINTH ANNUAL REPORT TO CONGRESS ON HIGH-PRIORITY EVIDENCE GAPS FOR CLINICAL PREVENTIVE SERVICES" (2019)

- Mental health and substance use
    - Preventive interventions for perinatal depression
    - Screening and behavioral counseling interventions for unhealthy alcohol use in adolescents and adults
    - Primary care interventions for tobacco use prevention and cessation in children and adolescents
    - Screening by asking about drug use for illicit drug use, including nonmedical use of prescription drugs, in adolescents and adults
- Violence prevention
    - Screening for intimate partner violence, elder abuse, and abuse of vulnerable adults
    - Interventions for child maltreatment

"EIGHTH ANNUAL REPORT TO CONGRESS ON HIGH-PRIORITY EVIDENCE GAPS FOR CLINICAL PREVENTIVE SERVICES" (2018)

- Cancer prevention
    - Screening for cervical cancer, especially among diverse populations
    - Screening for prostate cancer, especially among African American men and men with a family history
    - Screening and behavioral counseling for skin cancer
- Cardiovascular health
    - Screening for atrial fibrillation with electrocardiography
    - Screening for cardiovascular disease risk with electrocardiography
    - Risk assessment for cardiovascular disease with nontraditional risk factors
    - Screening for peripheral artery disease and cardiovascular disease risk assessment with the Ankle-Brachial Index

"SEVENTH ANNUAL REPORT TO CONGRESS ON HIGH-PRIORITY EVIDENCE GAPS FOR CLINICAL PREVENTIVE SERVICES" (2017)

- Topics where more research is needed
    - Screening for celiac disease
    - Screening for obstructive sleep apnea in adults

  - Screening for gynecologic conditions with pelvic examination
  - Vision screening in children younger than age 3 years
  - Statin use for the primary prevention of cardiovascular disease in adults age 76 years and older
- Evidence gaps relating to specific populations
  - Screening for breast cancer in African American women
  - Screening for prostate cancer in African American men
  - Screening for illicit drug use in children and adolescents
  - Screening for hearing loss in older adults

"SIXTH ANNUAL REPORT TO CONGRESS ON HIGH-PRIORITY EVIDENCE GAPS FOR CLINICAL PREVENTIVE SERVICES" (2016)

- Topics where further research is needed
  - Screening for autism spectrum disorder in young children
  - Screening for chlamydia and gonorrhea in men
  - Tobacco smoking cessation (electronic nicotine delivery systems) in adults
  - Vitamin supplementation (nutrients and multivitamins) to prevent cancer and cardiovascular disease
  - Screening for skin cancer in adults
- Evidence gaps relating to specific populations
  - Screening for breast cancer in African American women
  - Screening for cervical cancer in Hispanic and African American women
  - Screening for colorectal cancer in African Americans and American Indians/Alaska Natives

"FIFTH ANNUAL REPORT TO CONGRESS ON HIGH-PRIORITY EVIDENCE GAPS FOR CLINICAL PREVENTIVE SERVICES" (2015)

- Screening for intimate partner violence, illicit drug use, and mental health conditions
- Screening for thyroid dysfunction
- Screening for vitamin D deficiency and vitamin D and calcium supplementation to prevent fractures; screening for osteoporosis
- Screening for cancer
- Implementing clinical preventive services

"FOURTH ANNUAL REPORT TO CONGRESS ON HIGH-PRIORITY EVIDENCE GAPS FOR CLINICAL PREVENTIVE SERVICES" (2014)

- Evidence gaps relating to the care of children and adolescents
  - Mental health conditions and substance abuse
  - Obesity and cardiovascular health
  - Behavior and development
  - Infectious diseases
  - Cancer prevention
  - Injury and child maltreatment
  - Vision disorders

"THIRD ANNUAL REPORT TO CONGRESS ON HIGH-PRIORITY EVIDENCE GAPS FOR CLINICAL PREVENTIVE SERVICES" (2013)

- Evidence gaps related to the care of older adults
  - Screening for cognitive impairment and dementia
  - Screening for physical and mental well-being of older adults
  - Preventing falls and fractures
  - Screening for vision and hearing problems
  - Avoiding the unintended harms of medical procedures and testing in older adults

"SECOND ANNUAL REPORT TO CONGRESS ON HIGH-PRIORITY EVIDENCE GAPS FOR CLINICAL PREVENTIVE SERVICES" (2012)

- Topics where further research is needed
  - Screening for chronic kidney disease
  - Screening for cervical cancer with human papillomavirus (HPV) tests
  - Screening for prostate cancer
- Evidence gaps relating to specific populations
  - Screening for chronic kidney disease in African American adults
  - Screening for prostate cancer in African American men
  - Counseling about sun-protective behaviors in families with children under age 10 to reduce the risk for skin cancer

"FIRST ANNUAL REPORT TO CONGRESS ON HIGH-PRIORITY EVIDENCE GAPS FOR CLINICAL PREVENTIVE SERVICES" (2011)

- Screening tests
  - Screening for coronary heart disease with new and old technologies
  - Screening for colorectal cancer with new modalities
  - Screening for hepatitis C
  - Screening for hip dysplasia in newborns
- Behavioral interventions
  - Moderate to low-intensity counseling for obesity
  - Interventions in primary care to prevent child abuse and neglect
  - Screening for illicit drug use in primary care

F

U.S. Preventive Service Task Force Research Needs Statements from I Statements Issued Between 2017 and 2021

Gestational Diabetes: Screening (USPSTF, 2021a)

August 10, 2021

The U.S. Preventive Services Task Force (USPSTF) identified several gaps in the evidence where more research is needed. These include

- Studies (specifically randomized controlled trials [RCTs]) on the effect of screening for gestational diabetes and health outcomes.
- Studies examining the benefits and harms of screening for and treatment of gestational diabetes in pregnant persons before 24 weeks of gestation.
- Studies reporting on the effects of screening for gestational diabetes on populations defined by race/ethnicity, age, and other relevant socioeconomic factors.
- Studies examining how health outcomes differ by screening strategy (1- versus 2-step testing and various thresholds for gestational diabetes, fasting plasma glucose level, and HbA_{1c} concentration).
- Greater consistency in both the diagnostic criteria and outcome definitions used in studies.
- More studies that report on maternal health outcomes, especially hypertension and preeclampsia.
- Studies focusing on longer-term outcomes (i.e., obesity, impaired fasting glucose) for both pregnant persons and children.
- Studies on potential harms of screening and treatment (i.e., anxiety, hospital experience, and cesarean delivery).

Vitamin D Deficiency in Adults: Screening (USPSTF, 2021d)

April 13, 2021

More studies are needed that address the following areas:

- More research is needed to determine whether total serum 25(OH)D levels are the best measure of vitamin D deficiency and whether the best measure of vitamin D deficiency varies by subgroups defined by race, ethnicity, or sex.
- More research is needed to determine the cutoff that defines vitamin D deficiency and whether that cutoff varies by specific clinical outcome or by subgroups defined by race, ethnicity, or sex.
- When vitamin D deficiency is better defined, studies on the benefits and harms of screening for vitamin D deficiency will be helpful.

Hearing Loss in Older Adults: Screening (USPSTF, 2021c)

March 23, 2021

More studies are needed that address the following areas:

- The benefit of screening for and treatment of hearing loss in asymptomatic adults on health outcomes, such as quality of life and function, not just on hearing aid use or quality of hearing.
- The potential harms of screening and treatment, such as false-positive results and overtreatment.
- Consistent use of definitions of hearing loss to improve certainty about the accuracy of screening tests.
- The general adult population, as well as diverse subpopulations.
- The role of over-the-counter assistive hearing devices compared with prescription amplification devices.
- Screening tools that identify not just adults with hearing loss by audiometry definition criteria, but adults with unrecognized hearing loss that would benefit (the most) from amplification.

Tobacco Smoking Cessation in Adults, Including Pregnant Persons: Interventions (USPSTF, 2021b)

January 19, 2021

The greatest research needs are to gain a better understanding of the effectiveness of e-cigarettes for smoking cessation, as well as potential short- and long-term harms of e-cigarette use, and to understand whether there are effective pharmacotherapy options for pregnant persons.

- E-cigarettes: Given the potential negative effect that increasing e-cigarette use in youth is having on overall tobacco control efforts, there is an urgent need for research that provides both a clearer understanding of whether e-cigarettes may increase adult tobacco smoking cessation, as well as the potential harms of e-cigarette use as a tobacco product. Future research on e-cigarettes for smoking cessation in adults should address the following:

 - Studies must be well-designed RCTs that compare e-cigarette interventions with placebo, as well as established, effective combinations of pharmacotherapy and behavioral support.
 - Studies should be adequately powered to detect differences in continued smoking abstinence rates at 6 months or more.
 - Given the high rate of continued e-cigarette use after smoking cessation, research on both the short- and long-term harms of e-cigarette use is needed, as well as the harms in dual users of e-cigarettes and conventional cigarettes. More research is needed on smoking relapse rates in adults who have used e-cigarettes for smoking cessation and how to help with cessation of e-cigarette use once smoking abstinence has been achieved.
 - Given the rapidly evolving landscape of e-cigarettes, trials should include current generations of e-cigarettes. Additionally, to successfully conduct these types of studies, standardization of how to quantify e-cigarette use and levels of nicotine exposure from e-cigarettes is needed.
 - More research is needed to understand the patterns of e-cigarette use in youth and the risk factors for their transition from e-cigarette use to conventional cigarette smoking.
 - More research is also needed to better understand patterns of e-cigarette use in pregnant persons and potential harms of e-cigarette use to both pregnant persons and their offspring.
 - More research is needed on understanding how to help adults quit e-cigarettes.

- Pharmacotherapy in pregnant persons: Although behavioral counseling interventions have been found to be effective in improving smoking cessation during pregnancy, additional research is needed on pharmacotherapy options, in particular NRT, for pregnant persons for whom behavioral counseling interventions alone are not effective.
  - Larger studies adequately powered to detect an effect on both smoking cessation rates (during pregnancy and postpartum) and changes in perinatal and child health outcomes are needed.
  - A better understanding of why adherence rates to NRT during pregnancy is so low would also be helpful.

Although the benefits of behavioral counseling interventions and pharmacotherapy in nonpregnant adults and the benefits of behavioral counseling interventions in pregnant adults are well established, additional research on effective components of behavioral counseling and who to target specific interventions to would be informative. More research on newer modalities and remotely delivered interventions (mobile phone apps, Internet-based interventions) would also be helpful. Additionally, the effectiveness of interventions for cessation of other forms of tobacco and whether interventions need to be tailored to individual tobacco product types are also needed. Last, more research is needed on interventions to prevent relapse of tobacco use.

High Blood Pressure in Children and Adolescents: Screening (USPSTF, 2020c)

November 10, 2020

There are several critical evidence gaps in understanding the potential net benefit of screening for high blood pressure in childhood and adolescence. Studies are needed that provide more information on

- The test accuracy of blood pressure measurements with sphygmomanometers or oscillometric automated devices and establishing thresholds for hypertension for 24-hour ambulatory monitoring.
- The application of new thresholds for determining abnormal blood pressure to existing data sets and testing the validity of these thresholds.
- The benefits and harms of long-term pharmacologic treatment. These studies should have long-term follow-up of several months or years across various age groups because benefits and harms of treatments may be age dependent and hypertension in children may be self-limiting.
- The benefits and harms of screening and treatment should also include children at increased risk, such as Black and Hispanic/Latino populations.
- The long-term natural history of hypertension in children and the spontaneous resolution of hypertension.
- The associations among childhood hypertension, adulthood hypertension, and surrogate measures of cardiovascular disease in childhood and adulthood, as well as adulthood clinical cardiovascular disease.
- The harms of medications, long-term adherence with treatment, and the effect of individual components of multifactorial interventions.

Unhealthy Drug Use: Screening (USPSTF, 2020f)

June 9, 2020

The USPSTF identified important gaps related to screening for unhealthy drug use. To fill these gaps, the USPSTF needs more evidence from well-designed studies that further evaluate the following:

- The effectiveness of screening and interventions for drug use in adolescents.
- The optimal screening interval for detecting unhealthy drug use.
- The accuracy of screening tools for detecting nonmedical use of prescription drugs, including opioids.
- Strategies to improve access to pharmacotherapy and psychosocial interventions for persons with various types of drug use disorders.

- The harms that occur when the result of screening is punitive.
- The benefits and harms of providing prophylactic prescriptions for naloxone "rescue therapy" to patients in whom opioid misuse or opioid use disorders are detected after primary care screening.

Illicit Drug Use in Children, Adolescents, and Young Adults: Primary Care–Based Interventions (USPSTF, 2020d)

May 26, 2020

The USPSTF identified several gaps in the evidence where more research is needed:

- There was promising evidence that interventions could be effective in preventing cannabis use specifically; however, the benefit to harm ratio could not be determined because of a lack of studies reporting harms. Future research on cannabis prevention that deliberately addresses both benefits and harms is needed.
- There was minimal reporting on health, social, or legal outcomes and significant heterogeneity in reporting on drug use outcomes. Standardization of outcome measurement across trials would greatly strengthen the evidence base and improve the ability to pool data.
- Several interventions such as the Familias Unidas program (a family-based intervention program focusing on Hispanic youth) and interventions that included clinician training, education, personal coaching, and continuous quality improvement components showed promise in reducing illicit drug use. More studies are needed that replicate and further refine these interventions.
- There was no evidence on preventing or reducing illicit drug use in children younger than 10 years and limited evidence in young adults (aged 18–25 years). More data are needed on the benefits and harms of interventions in these age groups.
- Technology-based interventions such as text-based messaging, smartphone apps, games, web-based interventions, and social media have the potential for wide reach, although there are limited data about their effectiveness. More studies of implementation of these types of interventions is needed, specifically among families referred from primary care, to determine their uptake and effectiveness.

Tobacco Use in Children and Adolescents: Primary Care Interventions (USPSTF, 2020e)

April 28, 2020

More studies are needed to identify effective interventions to help children and adolescents who use tobacco products to quit.

- Larger, adequately powered studies and studies of new behavioral counseling interventions for cessation are needed.
    - These studies should report tobacco cessation outcomes at 6 months or later and should also provide information on components of the behavioral counseling intervention provided in the study (such as intensity of delivery, frequency of contacts, content and type of counseling or materials provided, delivery setting of studies, and training of persons delivering the intervention).
- More studies are needed that evaluate the benefits and harms of medications to help youth with tobacco cessation.
- More research is needed on interventions tailored specifically to prevent initiation of use and promote cessation of e-cigarette use in youth. The landscape of e-cigarette devices is rapidly evolving, so research in this area is challenged by the need to be timely, flexible, and comprehensive.
- More research is also needed on interventions tailored specifically to prevent initiation of use and promote cessation of other types of tobacco (such as, but not limited to, cigars and smokeless tobacco) and interventions tailored to subpopulations with elevated tobacco use rates (such as African American youth, Native American/Alaska Native youth, LGBTQ youth, and youth with mental illness).

Bacterial Vaginosis in Pregnant Persons to Prevent Preterm Delivery: Screening (USPSTF, 2020a)

April 7, 2020

More studies are needed to evaluate screening for and treatment of asymptomatic bacterial vaginosis in pregnant persons at increased risk for preterm delivery. These studies should

- Include pregnant persons with a history of prior preterm delivery, as well as other risk factors for preterm delivery, such as cervical insufficiency, multifetal gestation, young or advanced maternal age, low maternal body mass index (<20), and African American, Native Hawaiian/Other Pacific Islander, or American Indian/Alaska Native race/ethnicity.
- Be adequately powered to detect a reduction of all-cause preterm delivery prior to 37 weeks' gestation.

If a reduction in preterm delivery is found with treatment of asymptomatic bacterial vaginosis in pregnant persons at increased risk for preterm delivery, then additional research is needed on ways to better identify persons at increased risk for preterm delivery. Additionally, given the biochemical and hormonal changes that occur during pregnancy, further studies of bacterial vaginosis screening tests in pregnant persons are needed to confirm test accuracy in this population.

Cognitive Impairment in Older Adults: Screening (USPSTF, 2020b)

February 25, 2020

- More research is needed on the effect of screening and early detection of cognitive impairment (MCI and mild to moderate dementia) on important patient, caregiver, and societal outcomes, including decision making, advance planning, and caregiver outcomes.
- The body of evidence on screening and interventions for cognitive impairment would benefit from more consistent definitions and reporting of outcomes to allow comparisons across trials, especially from trials with longer-term follow-up.
- Studies are needed of the effects of caregiver or patient–caregiver dyad interventions on delay or prevention of institutionalization, and the effects of delay in institutionalization on caregivers.
- Research is needed on treatments that clearly affect the long-term clinical course of cognitive impairment. It is also important that studies on screening and interventions for cognitive impairment report harms and reasons for attrition of trial participants.

Abdominal Aortic Aneurysm: Screening (USPSTF, 2019a)

December 10, 2019

Addressing several key research gaps could help inform the benefit of screening for AAA in U.S.-based populations[1]:

- Although evidence shows that women who smoke or have a family history are at increased risk for AAA compared with nonsmoking women without a family history, evidence is insufficient that screening this population confers a net benefit. Ideally, appropriately powered RCTs among women with risk factors could answer these critical gaps in the evidence on screening for AAA. In the absence of new trial data, high-quality, well-calibrated modeling studies based on reliable data on the harms and benefits of screening in women who smoke or in men and women with a family history of AAA may be informative.
- Well-conducted cohort studies examining rescreening benefits (including growth rates and health outcomes) are needed for persons who initially screen negative for AAA to determine the benefit and timing of additional screening ultrasonography.
- External validation of risk prediction models that have already been developed will allow policy makers to assess their value for making more individualized screening recommendations.
- Epidemiologic studies on the current prevalence of AAA in the United States, including in subpopulations, would help inform the applicability of older population-based screening trials to the current U.S. population.
- Well-designed studies, RCTs, or registry data on the thresholds for repair of AAA in women may inform the benefits and harms of screening in

women, as evidence suggests that AAAs in women may rupture at a smaller size than in men.

- Studies examining systems approaches to improving implementation of evidence-based AAA screening in the United States are needed.
- Studies examining the efficacy of screening and treatment in diverse populations (e.g., older adults, women, and racial/ethnic groups) are needed to inform the need for specific recommendations in subpopulations of Americans.

Elevated Blood Lead Levels in Children and Pregnant Women: Screening (USPSTF, 2019b)

April 16, 2019

Research is needed to better inform decisions about screening for elevated blood lead levels in children and pregnant women, such as the development of validated questionnaires to identify at-risk populations most likely to benefit from screening. Studies reporting intermediate and health outcomes, outcomes in newborns, and harms in women and infants are needed, as well as studies evaluating effective interventions for reducing blood lead levels in pregnant women. Research is also needed to evaluate the effectiveness of treatments for elevated blood lead levels in trials with adequate sample sizes to inform treatment strategies. However, randomized trials may not always be appropriate for screening and environmental interventions because of ethical issues. Well-designed research studies are needed on the benefits of nutritional supplementation in reducing blood lead levels in children. Research on newer approaches to detecting elevated blood lead levels, such as point-of-care testing, that include intraindividual and interlaboratory reliability would be useful for assessing screening strategies in children and pregnant women. Different sources of lead exposure that are now emerging in at-risk communities are not well incorporated into current screening questionnaires. Research on screening and prevention in these populations remains limited. Additional research is needed to validate these potential risk factors in specific geographic locations and among at-risk populations.

Child Maltreatment: Interventions (USPSTF, 2018e)

November 27, 2018

The USPSTF recognizes the importance of this serious health problem and calls for the prioritization of research to address gaps in numerous areas related to child maltreatment. There is limited evidence supporting the use of risk-assessment instruments to identify children at risk of maltreatment. Further research to determine effective methods for clinicians to identify children at increased risk should be a priority.

Although most studies included home visitation, there was significant heterogeneity in study design and outcome measurements. Standardization of outcome measurement across trials would greatly strengthen the evidence base and improve the ability to pool data. Additionally, research on home visitation should base interventions on proven and well-designed theoretical models. Without this type of contextual information, it will be difficult to interpret whether inventions are successful and, if so, how those interventions worked. When investigating interventions and outcomes, the inclusion of diverse populations and settings would help improve the applicability of study findings. These would include families with known risk factors for child maltreatment (e.g., history of substance abuse in the home) and settings with limited access to social services. In addition, future research is needed to determine whether there are unintended harms from risk assessment and preventive interventions.

Unhealthy Alcohol Use in Adolescents and Adults: Screening and Behavioral Counseling Interventions (USPSTF, 2018j)

November 13, 2018

The USPSTF has identified several research gaps. Although difficult, conducting a trial with an unscreened comparison group to understand the population-level effects of screening in primary care settings would be valuable. More direct evidence is needed on the harms associated with screening and behavioral interventions. The USPSTF found a preliminary study that evaluated the USAUDIT and USAUDIT-C, recent U.S. adaptations of the AUDIT and AUDIT-C. Further test performance studies are needed to confirm their accuracy in identifying unhealthy alcohol use in various populations. More evidence on important clinical outcomes is needed, such as longer-term morbidity, mortality, health care utilization, and social and legal outcomes. Trials designed a priori to report subgroup effects in diverse populations (e.g., by age, sex, race/ethnicity, or baseline severity) would be useful. Limited evidence is available to assess the effects of screening and behavioral counseling in adolescents, and high-quality studies specifically addressing this population are needed. In addition, studies in adolescents are often conducted in school settings, which may not translate to primary care settings. More studies of adolescents in primary care settings are needed.

Intimate Partner Violence, Elder Abuse, and Abuse of Vulnerable Adults: Screening (USPSTF, 2018f)

October 23, 2018

There are several key research gaps related to IPV. The USPSTF recognizes that a significant body of evidence is lacking for men. The CDC has conducted studies demonstrating the prevalence and importance of IPV in men; however, there is a lack of research on screening and interventions to prevent IPV in men. Research is needed in all areas related to the accuracy of screening tools for men, and trials are needed that examine the effectiveness (benefits and harms) of screening and interventions for IPV in the primary care setting in men without recognized signs and symptoms of abuse.

More research is also needed on the most effective characteristics of ongoing support services for reducing IPV. In particular, more RCTs that compare the benefits and harms of screening (plus ongoing support services or referral for women who screen positive) versus no screening are needed, where support services may include more frequent and intensive interventions such as home visits, cognitive behavioral therapy, or other forms that address multiple risk factors. These studies should evaluate the optimal duration, format, and method of delivery.

Trials of ongoing support services should enroll women of all ages, including nonpregnant women and women beyond reproductive age. These trials will help with understanding the types of postscreening, ongoing support services that can be most effective, and the patients for whom they are most effective.

More research is also needed in all areas related to the accuracy of screening tools in the primary care setting for elder abuse and abuse of vulnerable adults when there are no recognized signs and symptoms of abuse. High-quality RCTs are also needed on the effectiveness (benefits and harms) of screening and interventions in the primary care setting to prevent such abuse.

Atrial Fibrillation: Screening with Electrocardiography (USPSTF, 2018b)

August 7, 2018

The connection between atrial fibrillation and stroke is well established, as is the existence of undiagnosed atrial fibrillation, especially among older adults. Randomized trials enrolling asymptomatic persons that directly compare screening with usual care and that assess both health outcomes and harms are needed to understand the balance of benefits and harms of screening for atrial fibrillation. Other research needs include understanding how to best optimize the accuracy of ECG interpretation. Although the evidence review for this recommendation statement focused on screening with ECG, the effectiveness of newer technologies capable of assessing pulse and heart rhythm as potential screening strategies should be evaluated. In addition, as ECG and other technologies (e.g., AliveCOR Kardia system [AliveCor Inc.], discussed in the context of the REHEARSE-AF trial below) are used to record heart activity for longer periods and thus are able to detect shorter episodes of arrhythmia, understanding the stroke risk associated with brief episodes of subclinical atrial fibrillation, and the potential benefit of anticoagulation therapy if risk is significant, is another important research need.

Several ongoing trials may help to fill these evidence gaps. The STROKE-STOP study (NLM, 2012) randomized 28,768 Swedish adults aged 75–76 years to be invited or not invited for screening, first with 12-lead ECG and then intermittently with a single handheld lead over 2 weeks. The primary outcome is stroke incidence. The SCREEN-AF study (NLM, 2015) randomized more than 800 participants to a 2-week ambulatory ECG patch monitor or usual care. The primary outcome is new diagnosis of ECG-confirmed atrial fibrillation or flutter, but clinical events are included as secondary outcomes. The IDEAL-MD study (NLM, 2014) randomized 16,000 adults older than 65 years to screening with a single-lead ECG device or usual care. The primary outcome is new diagnosis of atrial fibrillation over 1 year; secondary outcomes include major cardiovascular events and all-cause mortality. Last, the Detecting and Diagnosing Atrial Fibrillation (D_2AF) study (University Medical Center Utrecht, n.d.) is a cluster randomized trial that compares different approaches to case-finding among adults 65 years and older. The primary outcome is the difference in detection rate of new atrial fibrillation cases over 1 year compared with usual care; however, the study does not include clinical outcomes.

Peripheral Artery Disease and Cardiovascular Disease: Screening and Risk Assessment with the Ankle-Brachial Index (USPSTF, 2018h)

July 10, 2018

Large, population-based, randomized trials of screening versus no screening are needed to determine whether screening for PAD with the ABI improves clinical outcomes. One ongoing study in Denmark has published preliminary results; however, that study limited enrollment to men aged 65–74 years and included screening for abdominal aortic aneurysm and high blood pressure, making it difficult to evaluate the benefit of screening with the ABI alone.[2] Two other ongoing trials that include the ABI as part of a screening bundle may have the same limitation (Betriu et al., 2016; Diederichsen et al., 2015). Future studies, in addition to isolating the effect of individual tests, should address the population of persons at potentially increased risk for PAD who are not already receiving interventions to reduce cardiovascular risk, because this is the population most likely to benefit from an additional screening intervention. Studies of screening with the ABI and interventions to stop disease progression in the lower limbs in more diverse populations (e.g., women, racial/ethnic minorities, or persons with a lower socioeconomic status) and populations at high risk (i.e., persons with diabetes) would also be valuable.

Cardiovascular Disease: Risk Assessment with Nontraditional Risk Factors (USPSTF, 2018d)

July 10, 2018

A substantial number of studies demonstrate an association between the ABI, hsCRP level, and CAC score and cardiovascular outcomes, so additional association studies are unlikely to add more information. Similarly, studies assessing nontraditional risk factors in isolation are of limited value, given that current treatment recommendations are based on risk assessment with the Framingham Risk Score or Pooled Cohort Equations. Good-quality studies comparing traditional risk assessment with traditional risk assessment plus the ABI, hsCRP level, or CAC scores are needed to measure the effect of adding nontraditional risk factors on clinical decision thresholds and patient outcomes (CVD events and mortality). Studies are especially needed in more diverse populations (women, racial/ethnic minorities, persons of lower socioeconomic status), in whom assessment of nontraditional risk factors may help address the shortcomings of traditional risk models. In addition, well-designed prospective studies reflective of real-world practice are needed to identify the downstream effects of CAC score on additional testing and procedures.

Osteoporosis to Prevent Fractures: Screening (USPSTF, 2018g)

June 26, 2018

The majority of reviewed studies focused on women. Treatment trials that focus on or include men and report on fracture outcomes (rather than BMD) as well as harms are needed. More studies are also needed that evaluate the direct effect of screening for osteoporosis (either with BMD or clinical risk assessment tools) on fracture outcomes. Additional research is needed to determine whether clinical risk assessment tools alone (without BMD) could help identify patients at risk of fractures and help guide decisions to initiate medications to prevent fractures. The development of prognostic models incorporating age, baseline BMD, and hormone replacement therapy use[27,28] may also help identify optimal screening intervals.

Cardiovascular Disease Risk: Screening with Electrocardiography (USPSTF, 2018c)

June 12, 2018

A considerable number of studies have reported hazard ratios and other measures of association between ECG changes and cardiovascular outcomes, so additional studies of this nature are unlikely to advance the field. Studies are needed that assess the incremental value of adding ECG to current CVD risk assessment tools or instruments to directly inform decision making; studies that examine patient outcomes would be most useful. Failing that, studies are needed that assess the added value of ECG for risk reclassification across clinically relevant risk thresholds. Any study of CVD risk assessment should also evaluate the harms associated with assessment as well as those related to additional testing and treatment. Studies that measure risk reclassification should report total, event, and nonevent Net Reclassification Indices, with corresponding confidence intervals, as well as measures of calibration and discrimination.

Vitamin D, Calcium, or Combined Supplementation for the Primary Prevention of Fractures in Community-Dwelling Adults: Preventive Medication (USPSTF, 2018k)

April 17, 2018

Research is needed to determine whether daily supplementation with doses greater than 400 IU of vitamin D and greater than 1000 mg of calcium reduces fracture incidence in postmenopausal women and in older men. Prospective studies should assess the potential benefits of vitamin D and calcium supplementation in premenopausal women on fracture incidence later in life. Studies need to be adequately powered and should evaluate consistent fracture outcomes. Studies are also needed to evaluate the effects of vitamin D supplementation on diverse populations. Because white women have the highest risk for osteoporotic fractures, most fracture prevention studies have been conducted in this population, and it is difficult to extrapolate results to nonwhite populations. In addition, more studies evaluating the potential harms of supplementation are needed, particularly studies on calcium and potential adverse cardiovascular outcomes.

Skin Cancer Prevention: Behavioral Counseling (USPSTF, 2018i)
March 20, 2018

A better understanding of the effectiveness of counseling on the use of sun protection behaviors in adults 25 years and older is needed to address the key evidence gap on counseling for this age group. Research that evaluates the association between UV exposure during adulthood and skin cancer risk would also be valuable.

In addition, studies regarding the effectiveness of counseling persons without a fair skin type are lacking. Ideally, research studies would provide measurements of sun exposure, sunburn, precursor skin lesions, and cancer among large trial populations, with an emphasis on behaviors and health outcomes among persons who receive an intervention focused on sun protection behaviors. Such studies would also assess whether these behaviors continue after trial completion. These cohorts should include populations with diverse skin colors and should include adolescents, young adults, and preschool-aged children and their parents. These studies may be used to further develop technologies and vehicles for administering relevant interventions for behavior change in the primary care setting, especially among nonwhite persons, young adults, and persons who practice indoor or outdoor tanning. Further evidence is needed to assess the balance of benefits and harms of counseling adults about skin self-examination to prevent skin cancer and premature death.

Adolescent Idiopathic Scoliosis: Screening (USPSTF, 2018a)
January 9, 2018

The USPSTF identified several research gaps. Prospective, controlled screening studies that allow for comparison of screened and nonscreened populations and different screening settings, personnel, and procedures are needed. Good-quality studies with prospective identification of cohorts at the time of diagnosis (e.g., from geographical areas with and without routine screening for adolescent idiopathic scoliosis) or treatment (e.g., treated versus observed cohorts) for the purpose of long-term follow-up are important. High-quality studies on the potential harms of screening and treatment are also needed. Additional studies to help determine whether individual characteristics (e.g., body mass index) may influence response to bracing treatment would be helpful. Studies on long-term outcomes are needed and should stratify results by degree of spinal curvature at diagnosis and at skeletal maturity. Better information on long-term outcomes such as pulmonary disorders, disability, back pain, psychological effects, cosmetic issues, and quality of life would be helpful. Good-quality studies on treatment with exercise, bracing, and surgery among screen-detected patients are needed. Studies conducted in primary care settings are also needed.

Vision in Children Ages 6 Months to 5 Years: Screening (USPSTF, 2017d)

September 5, 2017

The USPSTF identified several gaps in the evidence. Well-designed trials are needed to better understand the effects of screening versus no screening, the optimal age for initiation of screening, and appropriate screening intervals. Additional studies are needed to determine the best screening approach and most favorable combinations of screening tests in primary care. There is also a need for studies that examine the benefits and harms of vision screening and treatment in children younger than 3 years and the long-term benefits and harms of preschool vision screening on health outcomes, such as quality of life, school performance, developmental trajectory, and functioning.

Celiac Disease: Screening (USPSTF, 2017a)

March 28, 2017

Studies that randomly assign participants to screening versus no screening and evaluate clinical outcomes are lacking. However, screening studies that target populations at increased risk for celiac disease are likely to be more informative than trials that target the general population, because of the higher prevalence of disease, and should be given higher priority. More information is needed about the accuracy of serologic testing in asymptomatic persons, particularly those with disease risk factors.

Treatment studies in screen-detected, asymptomatic persons are also needed to understand the effects of adherence to a gluten-free diet (compared with no dietary intervention), as well as the effects of immediate versus delayed dietary changes (i.e., at the time of screen-detected diagnosis versus when symptoms develop). Ideally, studies would report both short-term effects on symptoms and quality of life and long-term outcomes (e.g., osteoporotic fractures, cancer, and mortality). As for screening, treatment studies focused on asymptomatic persons at high risk for celiac disease who screen positive would be helpful for developing guidance for this population and may be faster and more efficient to complete than other study designs. More research is needed to better understand the natural history of positive serology in patients without histologic changes or with histologic confirmation but no symptoms. Also, treatment studies should report results stratified according to baseline histologic findings, given current uncertainty about the natural history of celiac disease in persons with mild histologic abnormalities.

Gynecological Conditions: Periodic Screening with the Pelvic Examination (USPSTF, 2017b)

March 7, 2017

The USPSTF recognizes that research on the effectiveness of the screening pelvic examination is difficult, given that multiple conditions could potentially be detected with this single preventive service. However, in reviewing the currently available evidence on the benefits and harms of performing screening pelvic examinations in asymptomatic adult women, the USPSTF identified the following critical evidence gaps. Studies evaluating the accuracy and effectiveness of screening pelvic examination to detect conditions other than ovarian cancer, bacterial vaginosis, genital herpes, and trichomoniasis are lacking. Studies reporting on the harms of screening with pelvic examination (including quantified psychological harms) in asymptomatic women in primary care are also lacking.

Studies reporting the effects of performing routine screening pelvic examinations on health outcomes such as all-cause mortality, disease-specific morbidity and mortality, quality of life, and psychological benefits and harms could help fill the gaps in the existing evidence and inform future USPSTF recommendations. Studies evaluating and quantifying harms are needed, as well as studies evaluating the potential effectiveness of risk assessment tools to determine which women might benefit from a pelvic examination. Research is needed to clarify which indications primary care clinicians are currently using the screening pelvic examination for in asymptomatic patients and which components of the pelvic examination are performed most frequently. Studies exploring women's attitudes toward pelvic examinations, the outcomes women value from these examinations, and how pelvic examinations affect women's decisions to seek and obtain care are also needed to clarify the potential benefits and harms of providing this preventive service.

Obstructive Sleep Apnea in Adults: Screening (USPSTF, 2017c)

January 24, 2017

The identification of valid and reliable clinical prediction tools that could accurately determine which asymptomatic persons (or persons with unrecognized symptoms) would benefit from further evaluation and testing for OSA is needed. In addition, studies that evaluate the effect of OSA treatments or interventions on health outcomes (e.g., all-cause and cardiovascular mortality, cardiovascular disease and cerebrovascular events, motor vehicle crashes, and cognitive impairment) that are adequately powered and have an appropriate length of follow-up are needed. Studies are also needed to evaluate whether improvement in AHI (for mild to severe OSA) leads to improvement in health outcomes. These represent critical gaps in the current evidence base. The USPSTF has identified the need for further research on the effect on health outcomes of screening for OSA among asymptomatic persons in the general population, as well as the role of sleepiness in determining health outcomes. More data on the natural history of mild OSA are also needed, in particular the rates of progression from mild to severe OSA, the length of duration before progression, and the magnitude of benefit if OSA is identified and treated earlier.

REFERENCES

USPSTF (U.S. Preventive Services Task Force). 2017a. *Celiac disease: Screening*. https://www.uspreventiveservicestaskforce.org/uspstf/recommendation/celiac-disease-screening (accessed July 14, 2021).

USPSTF. 2017b. *Gynecological conditions: Periodic screening with the pelvic examination*. https://www.uspreventiveservicestaskforce.org/uspstf/recommendation/gynecological-conditions-screening-with-the-pelvic-examination (accessed August 17, 2021).

USPSTF. 2017c. *Obstructive sleep apnea in adults: Screening*. https://uspreventiveservicestaskforce.org/uspstf/recommendation/obstructive-sleep-apnea-in-adults-screening (accessed November 22, 2021).

USPSTF. 2017d. *Vision in children ages 6 months to 5 years: Screening*. https://www.uspreventiveservicestaskforce.org/uspstf/recommendation/vision-in-children-ages-6-months-to-5-years-screening (accessed August 17, 2021).

USPSTF. 2018a. *Adolescent idiopathic scoliosis: Screening*. https://www.uspreventiveservicestaskforce.org/uspstf/recommendation/adolescent-idiopathic-scoliosis-screening (accessed August 17, 2021).

USPSTF. 2018b. *Atrial fibrillation: Screening with electrocardiography*. https://www.uspreventiveservicestaskforce.org/uspstf/recommendation/atrial-fibrillation-screening-with-electrocardiography (accessed August 17, 2021).

USPSTF. 2018c. *Cardiovascular disease risk: Screening with electrocardiography*. https://www.uspreventiveservicestaskforce.org/uspstf/recommendation/cardiovascular-disease-risk-screening-with-electrocardiography (accessed August 17, 2021).

USPSTF. 2018d. *Cardiovascular disease: Risk assessment with nontraditional risk factors*. https://www.uspreventiveservicestaskforce.org/uspstf/recommendation/cardiovascular-disease-screening-using-nontraditional-risk-assessment (accessed August 17, 2021).

USPSTF. 2018e. *Child maltreatment: Interventions*. https://www.uspreventiveservicestaskforce.org/uspstf/recommendation/child-maltreatment-primary-care-interventions (accessed August 17, 2021).

USPSTF. 2018f. *Intimate partner violence, elder abuse, and abuse of vulnerable adults: Screening*. https://www.uspreventiveservicestaskforce.org/uspstf/recommendation/intimate-partner-violence-and-abuse-of-elderly-and-vulnerable-adults-screening (accessed August 17, 2021).

USPSTF. 2018g. *Osteoporosis to prevent fractures: Screening*. https://www.uspreventiveservicestaskforce.org/uspstf/recommendation/osteoporosis-screening (accessed August 17, 2021).

USPSTF. 2018h. *Peripheral artery disease and cardiovascular disease: Screening and risk assessment with the ankle-brachial index*. https://www.uspreventiveservicestaskforce.org/uspstf/recommendation/peripheral-artery-disease-in-adults-screening-with-the-ankle-brachial-index (accessed August 17, 2021).

USPSTF. 2018i. *Skin cancer prevention: Behavioral counseling*. https://www.uspreventiveservicestaskforce.org/uspstf/recommendation/skin-cancer-counseling (accessed August 17, 2021).

USPSTF. 2018j. *Unhealthy alcohol use in adolescents and adults: Screening and behavioral counseling interventions*. https://www.uspreventiveservicestaskforce.org/uspstf/recommendation/unhealthy-alcohol-use-in-adolescents-and-adults-screening-and-behavioral-counseling-interventions (accessed August 17, 2021).

USPSTF. 2018k. *Vitamin D, calcium, or combined supplementation for the primary prevention of fractures in community-dwelling adults: Preventive medication*. https://www.uspreventiveservicestaskforce.org/uspstf/recommendation/vitamin-d-calcium-or-combined-supplementation-for-the-primary-prevention-of-fractures-in-adults-preventive-medication (accessed August 17, 2021).

USPSTF. 2019a. *Abdominal aortic aneurysm: Screening.* https://www.uspreventiveservicestaskforce.org/uspstf/recommendation/abdominal-aortic-aneurysm-screening (accessed August 17, 2021).

USPSTF. 2019b. *Elevated blood lead levels in children and pregnant women: Screening.* https://www.uspreventiveservicestaskforce.org/uspstf/recommendation/elevated-blood-lead-levels-in-childhood-and-pregnancy-screening (accessed August 17, 2021).

USPSTF. 2020a. *Bacterial vaginosis in pregnant persons to prevent preterm delivery: Screening.* https://www.uspreventiveservicestaskforce.org/uspstf/recommendation/bacterial-vaginosis-in-pregnancy-to-prevent-preterm-delivery-screening (accessed August 17, 2021).

USPSTF. 2020b. *Cognitive impairment in older adults: Screening.* https://www.uspreventiveservicestaskforce.org/uspstf/recommendation/cognitive-impairment-in-older-adults-screening (accessed August 17, 2021).

USPSTF. 2020c. *High blood pressure in children and adolescents: Screening.* https://www.uspreventiveservicestaskforce.org/uspstf/recommendation/blood-pressure-in-children-and-adolescents-hypertension-screening (accessed August 17, 2021).

USPSTF. 2020d. *Illicit drug use in children, adolescents, and young adults: Primary care-based interventions.* https://www.uspreventiveservicestaskforce.org/uspstf/recommendation/drug-use-illicit-primary-care-interventions-for-children-and-adolescents (accessed August 17, 2021).

USPSTF. 2020e. *Tobacco use in children and adolescents: Primary care interventions.* https://www.uspreventiveservicestaskforce.org/uspstf/recommendation/tobacco-and-nicotine-use-prevention-in-children-and-adolescents-primary-care-interventions (accessed August 17, 2021).

USPSTF. 2020f. *Unhealthy drug use: Screening.* https://www.uspreventiveservicestaskforce.org/uspstf/recommendation/drug-use-illicit-screening (accessed August 17, 2021).

USPSTF. 2021a. *Gestational diabetes: Screening.* https://www.uspreventiveservicestaskforce.org/uspstf/recommendation/gestational-diabetes-screening (accessed August 17, 2021).

USPSTF. 2021b. *Hearing loss in older adults: Screening.* https://www.uspreventiveservicestaskforce.org/uspstf/recommendation/hearing-loss-in-older-adults-screening (accessed August 17, 2021).

USPSTF. 2021c. *Tobacco smoking cessation in adults, including pregnant persons: Interventions.* https://www.uspreventiveservicestaskforce.org/uspstf/recommendation/tobacco-use-in-adults-and-pregnant-women-counseling-and-interventions (accessed August 17, 2021).

USPSTF. 2021d. *Vitamin D deficiency in adults: Screening.* https://www.uspreventiveservicestaskforce.org/uspstf/recommendation/vitamin-d-deficiency-screening (accessed August 17, 2021).